MIND DIET PLAN

Feed Your Brain and keep it Younger!

By

Maya Bryce

The marks used shall be without consent, and the distribution of the mark shall be without the consent or support of the proprietor of the mark. All trademarks and trademarks within this book are just for explanation and are held clearly by the owners, who are not associated with this record.

TABLE OF CONTENTS

INTRODUCTION

Shedding pounds is the primary goal of most diet plans, especially when it comes to fad detoxes and cleanses. Nevertheless, not everyone on a diet wants to lose weight. Various diets can produce different results. You may consider trying your MIND diet, which is related to slower cognitive decline if you are hoping to improve your brain health and to prevent the start of Alzheimer's disease.

Alzheimer's disease — a gradual and debilitating memory loss and confusion-causing neurodegenerative disease — is affecting 5.8 million Americans and, according to the Alzheimer's Association, the most common type of dementia. In the United States, it is the sixth-largest cause of death, with one in 3 people dying of Alzheimer's or other forms of dementia.

Although there is no research linking the MIND diet with Alzheimer's reversal, there is plenty of evidence to support the connection between this dietary approach and disease prevention.

For years, doctors have said that what you eat will affect your heart 's health. There is now growing proof that the brain is the same. A recent research study at the Chicago Rush University Medical Center indicates that a diet plan that they have created – the correct MIND diet – will minimize the risk of Alzheimer's disease by as much as 53%.

For those who didn't stick entirely to the diet but "moderately well" followed, it decreased their risk of Alzheimer's by about a third.

Diet appears to be only one of 'many variables that play a role in deciding who gets the disease, 'said Martha Clare Morris, a diet epidemiologist, Ph.D., MIND lead author. Genetics and other factors, such as smoking, exercise, and education, are also significant. Nevertheless, the MIND diet helped slow down the deterioration rate and avoid Alzheimer's regardless of other risk factors.

The research, published in Alzheimer's & Dementia journal, analyzed over 900 people aged 58 to 98 who completed food questionnaires and were checked daily. Participants whose diets followed MIND guidelines closely were found to be 7.5 years younger with a degree of cognitive function.

The MIND diet splits its guidelines into 10 'brain safe food groups' to keep people from eating and 5 'unhealthy eating groups.'

The good health of the brain at any age partially depends on diet and food choices. Knowing the top brain-healthy foods (and foods from which they stay) will protect your brain in the long term.

It incorporates several elements of two other popular eating plans that have been shown to support heart health: the Mediterranean diet and the DASH diet. (MIND stands for Mediterranean-DASH neurodegenerative delay intervention.)

The MIND diet, however, also varied greatly from such strategies and was more effective than either in decreasing the risk of Alzheimer's disease.

The Mediterranean diet is the winner in terms of heart health. The DASH diet is the safest option for high blood pressure patients. These diets have shown a certain capacity to defend the brain against cognitive deterioration. Today, a diet consisting of brain-beneficial foods seems to help shield stroke survivors from dementia within ten years of their stroke.

The diet of Mediterranean-DASH for Neurodegenerative Delay (MIND) stresses the use of certain foods that have all been related to slower cognitive deterioration in medical trials. It also refers to food classes to be avoided based on adverse brain effects.

According to the founders of the MIND diet, ischemic stroke causes the brain to expand to 3.6 years of age per hour in which the stroke is untreated. This probably explains why stroke survivors are double the public dementia rate, and nearly 20% of stroke survivors develop dementia.

"The ability to alter these effects with a healthy diet has enormous consequences for thousands of people suffering from stroke every year," says nutritionist Kate Patton, RD.

USING FOOD AS MEDICINE

After the MIND diet started in 2015, cognitive deterioration in stable older adults has been shown to slow. A survey of healthy people in Chicago showed that those who followed the MIND diet were 7.5 years younger than those who followed the least diet.

Earlier this year at the International Stroke Conference, a study was presented comparing the Mediterranean, DASH, and MIND diets of stroke patients. This study found a 20-year difference in cognitive function among those who adhered to the MIND diet most and the least.

HOW THE MIND DIET IS UNIQUE?

All of the three diets promote meats, fish, whole grains, fresh fruit, and olive oil to be consumed and discourages salt. However, they have big variations.

The Mediterranean and DASH diets are different because the MIND diet reduces the type and quantity of fruit and vegetables to be eaten. The MIND diet states that berries are consumed and not fruits like the other diets. It does not even eat milk items, potatoes, or more than one fish meal a week.

The MIND diet recommends that green leafy vegetables and another vegetable be eaten each day, while the Mediterranean and DASH diets encourage the loading of all kinds of fruits and vegetables.

The MIND diet addresses restricting only cheese and butter in the case of dairy. The Mediterranean diet encourages moderate consumption of milk products and allows for eggs.

The MIND diet states that products with adverse brain influence are removed, such as red meat and processed foods, fried fast snacks, candies and pastries, butter, margarine stick, and whole-fat cheese.

Is it worth it?

The MIND diet must not be followed up to the letter. It should be used by its creators as a guideline to avoid and promote brain-friendly foods. Many people would consider the MIND diet enticing if they were confident that it would stave away dementia.

This confirmation will arrive by 2021 if clinical trial results for five years are announced. The study, supported by a grant from the National Institute for Aging, assesses the impact of the MIND diet on 600 elderly people, some of which are brain-scanned.

WHAT EXACTLY IS THE MIND DIET?

The latest dietary craze does not offer miracles or guarantees that belly fat will blow. Alternatively, it promises to reduce the risk of Alzheimer's, and it does indeed work.

Evidence has shown that the MIND diet can reduce the risk of Alzheimer's by 53 percent, depending on how closely you practice it. It is an effective preventive method, as one in three Canadians over the age of 85 suffer from Alzheimer's disease or some other form of dementia.

The dietary scheme is a blend of the Mediterranean diet with plant food and olive oil and DASH (Dietary Approaches to Stop Hypertension) low in saturated fat and sugar. These diets have already been related to the enhancement of heart health and cancer prevention, but together they can do good for your brain as well.

"This kind of diet is perfect for the whole body," says Rosie Schwartz, a registered nutritionist based in Toronto. She states that your dedication to the MIND diet should be lifelong, to get the best results for your brain and your general health. "The brain function loss doesn't happen immediately. Now we should look at our future."

THE HUMAN BRAIN AND THE FOOD WE EAT

Think about it. Think about it. It takes care of your thoughts and actions, your breathing, your pulse, and your senses – it works hard 24/7 even when you sleep. This means that your brain needs a constant fuel supply. The "heat" comes from the foods you consume — and all that makes a difference in that water. Simply put, what you eat directly affects your brain's structure, function, and mood.

Like a costly car, your brain will work best if only premium fuel is obtained. Eating high-quality, vitamin-containing foods, minerals, and antioxidants nourish the brain and protect it against oxidation stress, the "waste" produced by the use of oxygen in the body that can damage cells.

Unfortunately, just like an expensive vehicle, you will damage your brain if you drink anything but premium fuel. If "low-premium" fuel compounds (such as what you get from processed or refined foods) come into the brain, it is incapable of getting rid of these. For example, diets high in processed sugars are harmful to the brain. These also encourage inflammation and oxidative stress, in addition to weakening the body's insulin control. Many studies have found a correlation between a diet high in refined sugar and impaired brain function — and even worsening symptoms such as depressive mood disorders.

It's important. If the brain is without good nutrition or if free radicals or inflammatory cells circulate within the enclosed space of the brain, the effects should be predicted. What is surprising is that the medical field has not fully recognized the link between mood and food for many years.

Today, luckily, there are many implications and similarities about what you consume, how you feel and how you behave, and the kinds of bacteria that reside in your stomach, in the emerging field of nutritional psychiatry.

How the foods you eat affect how you feel

Serotonin is a neurotransmitter that assists sleep and appetite control, mediates mood, and reduces pain. Since about 95 percent of your serotonin is produced in your gastrointestinal tract, and you have a hundred million nerve cells or neurons lined with your gastrointestinal tract. It makes sense that your digestive system does not simply help digest food, but direct your emotions. However, the activity of these neurons — and the production of neurotransmitters such as serotonin — is profoundly affected by the thousands of 'healthy' bacteria throughout your intestinal microbiome. Such bacteria play an important part in your wellbeing. They protect the intestines and ensure they provide a strong barrier against toxins and bad bacteria, reduce inflammation, improve how well nutrients you absorb from your food and stimulate neural pathways between the intestines and the brain.

Studies have compared the modern "west" diet to "western" diets, such as the Mediterranean diet and traditional Japanese diets. They have shown that the risk of depression is 25 to 35% lower for those consuming a traditional diet. Scientists make this difference because these traditional diets often contain high amounts of vegetables, fruit, unprocessed grains, fish, and seafood and only contain modest quantities of meat and milk. These are also free of processed and refined foods and carbohydrates that make up the 'American' diet. Additionally, many of these unprocessed foods are fermented and therefore act as natural probiotics.

It sounds vague to you, but the theory that good bacteria affect not just what your gut digests and absorbs, but also the degree of inflammation around your body and your mood and energy level, increases researchers' traction.

Nutritional psychiatry: What does it mean for you?

Be aware of how many foods are consumed — not only right now, but the next day. Aim to eat a "clean" diet for two to three weeks – this means all refined food and sugar are cut off. See how you feel. Then gradually, one by one put food back into your diet and see how you feel.

When some "go clean," they cannot believe how much better both physically and emotionally, they feel and how much worse they feel when they reintroduce the foods that improve inflammation.

FOODS TO EAT ON A MIND DIET TO KEEP YOUR BRAIN YOUNG

To help sustain a healthy brain, include these foods that constitute the foundations of the MIND diet.

DARK LEAFY GREENS

Up to six servings per week. Such wholesome greens contain essential compounds that protect the brain, such as folate, phylloquinone, and lutein. For one study, which measured the leafy green consumption of adults up to 99 years of age for more than 4,5 years, researchers found only a little more than one serving of leafy green vegetables a day to retain brain capacity. The party that accomplished this goal had 11 years of younger memory and reasoning skills! It is so quick to incorporate these foods into food. At dinner, kindly add a little side salad, add kale to a smoothie, serve sautéed greens with an egg scramble and add rice, soups, and stew.

Other Veggies

Around one serving per day. Including leafy greens, the MIND diet (along with every balanced diet) emphasizes vegetables, and seek a different form of veggie every day. It doesn't have to be difficult. Place tomatoes and red pepper strips in sandwiches and fry them with broccoli, cauliflower, bring nice veggie noodles into pasta dinners (such as zucchini or carrot noodles) or just snack them with cherry tomatoes and hummus.

Nuts

Up to five servings per week. Nuts are filled with anti-inflammatory fats and other nutrients that help preserve the health of your brain as you grow old. One research looked at the eating habits of a large group of women for over a decade and found that women who consumed about five servings a week were brain-functioning two years younger than those who consumed the least nuts.

Sprinkle the nuts over the salads, garnish with winter soups, perfect yogurt and oatmeal, snack them, like energy bite and bars, or simply snack on a portion directly (around an ounce).

Pulses (beans and legumes)

More than three servings/week. By these plant protein forces, memory and perception are maintained better, and a second study also found that the opposite is true — lower intakes are related to a rise in cognitive declines. The MIND diet requires a total of three portions per week.

While you can increase your consumption by getting several meatless meals per week, along with a smaller portion of animal proteins, you can also have this vegetable protein. For starters, serve your turkey taco salad with some black beans and pine nuts, use hummus as a turkey sandwich, or serve a garlic white bean mash for a roast chicken or turkey side.

BERRIES

More than two servings/week. The antioxidants in berries called flavonoids are thought to help preserve the activity of your brain and decrease the chance of cognitive decline. The two-serving limit is quick to hit! To smoothies, milk, chia pudding, and cold cereal add fresh or non-sweetened frozen fruit. And serve some sweet berries with a Greek yogurt dollop and a sprinkling of nuts. Beers are also a good way to raise a salad in the season.

SEAFOOD

More than one serving/week. Although the Mediterranean diet and even our own Dietary Guidelines call for more seafood to be eaten (about twice a week), it can be easier to achieve the MIND dietary goal. Oily fish, such as salmon and sardines, provide particularly helpful anti-inflammatory omega-three fats. Canned wild tuna and salmon are easy options every day to meet your seafood needs.

Why is Fish Good for Your Brain?

Do you want to keep your brain shrinking as you grow old? Eat more fish. Eat more fish. This is the conclusion of a recent Neurology newspaper article. Based on the Framingham study in progress, researchers investigated the interrelationships between omega-3 levels in blood samples and brain size in over 1500 participants.

Omega-3s are unsaturated fats, especially fatty fish like salmon, sardine, and herring, found in the majority of fish. Omega-3s contains docosahexaenoic (DHA) and eicosapentaenoic (EPA) acid, as well as polyunsaturated (PUFA) fatty acids.

The study showed a mid-life lower level of DHA and EPA in red blood cells, as well as subtle signs of memory and cognitive decline, were correlated with accelerated brain aging and lower brain volume. The study adds to an increasing number of evidence that the lifestyle choices we now make will later impact our brain health.

POULTRY

More than two servings/week. This is another food choice that extremely versatile in the MIND diet. Opportunities are unless you are vegan or vegetarian, chicken and turkey are most likely to be already eaten. Such protein options for your brain are safer than red meat, such as beef, pork, and lamb.

WHOLE GRAINS

Up to three servings per day. Your brain uses a lot of energy — about 20% of the calories you eat are used to fuel your brain. And its main source of fuel is glucose, leading to carbohydrates breakdown. MIND, DASH, and Mediterranean diets emphasize the benefits of whole grains and science. In a survey of more than 5,000 people, a small amount of whole grain (and a higher intake of poorer foods, such as red meat) was correlated with a more severe cognitive decline. The research found significantly higher rates of cognitive performance over an 11years among those who followed the guidance of the DASH or Mediterranean diet. In particular, whole grains, nuts, and legumes were related to the better functioning of the brain.

Place your white bread sandwich over a whole grain, take brown rice over white rice and pick whole grain (including oatmeal) cereals and sides (such as quinoa).

EXTRA VIRGIN OLIVE OIL

The primary oil used by both the MIND and the Mediterranean diets is extra virgin olive oil, EVOO. Because quality EVOO has a distinct flavor, you can use more neutral avocado oil as a backup. Avocados' compounds have been related to increased blood pressure, blood sugar, and blood flow, all of which contribute to improving brain health.

WINE

One serving/day. Whether you love a glass of wine at night, the good news is that the MIND diet provides up to one glass of wine every day. While health guidelines encourage men to have two drinks a day, the MIND diet sticks with just one glass because older men do not metabolize alcohol just like younger men.

Because of its polyphenol content, wine is favored, which can provide some protection. Remember that while a glass of wine may be an excellent way to relax and maintain your brain capacity, more doesn't help and can increase your memory risk and other impairments.

Bonus: Dark chocolate

Although it is not included in the MIND diet, the influence of dark chocolate on brain health was also studied. Studies link dark chocolate, rich in antioxidant compounds known as flavonoids, to enhanced memory and better brain blood flow. Dark chocolate is also thought to increase brain neuroplasticity, which may enhance your brain's ability to learn as you grow old. Although sweets are consumed in moderation in a brain boost scheme, 70 or higher dark chocolate is a good choice if you eat them.

FOODS TO LIMIT OR AVOID TO KEEP YOUR MEMORY SHARP AND REDUCE YOUR RISK OF ALZHEIMER'S

Many foods help to keep your brain healthy, and others can also raise the risk of cognitive impairment and certain brain disorders. The MIND diet has only been ranked number 2 by the U.S. News & World Report would be especially beneficial to your brain. MIND stands for Mediterranean-DASH neurodegenerative delay intervention. It is based on the Mediterranean diet and the DASH diet, but it concentrates on foods that have been shown to enhance brain health.

Such five foods have been described by Martha Claire Morris, Sc. D., and her colleagues at the Rush University Medical Center as being related to impaired cognitive function and increased risk of Alzheimer's disease. For two factors, they are bad for the brain: either they're rich in saturated fat, which can cause inflammation and oxidative stress in your body, which can kill the brain cells, or are high in sugar. Intake of food filled with sugar interferes with insulin signaling, which is troublesome because insulin in the brain plays a significant role in education and memory.

Here's what the MIND diet will limit:

1. RED MEAT

Red meat has more fat than other sources of protein, such as poultry or tofu. One study also combined an increase in brain iron with an increased risk of Alzheimer's and suggested that high red meat intake could be a factor.

2. FRIED AND FAST FOOD

Many fried foods have unhealthy saturated fat levels, as do other fast foods.

3. WHOLE-FAT CHEESE

Less than one serving/week. Cheese saturated fat is high. While you might have learned that processed cheese that contains the metal aluminum and that may increase the risk of dementia, in recent years, it has been refuted that trace quantity of aluminum from food increases the risk of Alzheimer's.

4. BUTTER /MARGARINE

Less than one tablespoon/day. Butter is high in saturated fat, while vegetable oil, such as soybean oil for omega-6 fats, contains margarine. Too many omega-6s fats can cause inflammation to increase.

5. PASTRIES AND SWEETS

Fewer than five servings/week. These treats are also high in saturated fat and sugar. Sugar can also activate the recompense mechanism of your body, which makes you crave for more.

MIND DIET RELATION TO HEALTH ISSUES

MIND Diet May Decrease Oxidative Stress and Inflammation

The latest MIND diet research could not demonstrate exactly how it works. Nonetheless, scientists responsible for creating the diet claim that it can function by reducing oxidative stress and inflammation.

Oxidative stress is caused by large amounts of unstable molecules called free radicals in the body. This often causes cell damage. The brain is particularly vulnerable to such damage.

Inflammation is the natural reaction of the body to injury and infection. Nonetheless, if inflammation is not properly regulated, it can also be harmful and lead to many chronic diseases.

Oxidative stress and inflammation can be very harmful to the brain together. Several approaches to prevent and treat Alzheimer's disease have been based in recent years.

After the Mediterranean and DASH diets, oxidative stress and inflammation were lower.

Since the MIND diet is a hybrid of both diets, it is probably also the antioxidant and anti-inflammatory effects of the food that makes up the MIND diet.

Fruit antioxidants and vitamin E are known to support the brain's function by shielding the brain from oxidative stress in olive oils, green leafy vegetables, and nuts.

Also, omega-3 fatty acids present in fatty fish are known for their ability to decrease inflammation in the brain and for slow brain loss.

Researchers believe that the antioxidant and anti-inflammatory effects of foods promoted in the MIND diet can minimize dementia risk and delay brain damage that may occur during aging.

Anti-Inflammatory Foods Behind mind diet

We all want to age gracefully, particularly as a smaller risk of chronic diseases. However, the achievement of sufficient sleep, a healthy diet, sufficient physical activity, social interaction, and the reduction of stress, essential for achieving good health longer, remain unaffected for many.

For example, sleeping healthfully remains as vital as you grow old, but it appears to be harder to achieve. Fortunately, how you eat will improve your older years' health.

Benefits of Sleep Quality Can Be Improved with Diet

Although sleep focus usually concentrates on the number of hours of sleep, a team of researchers based in Athens (Greece) argued strongly in favor of a Mediterranean diet that increases sleep quality, thus distinguishing between sleep quality and sleep quantity.

In this longitudinal study, which was published in the journal Geriatrics & Gerontology International, researchers evaluated the duration and quality of sleep for 1639 adults 65 years old or older and their adherence in a Mediterranean diet based on self-registered questionnaires.

The researchers found that participants who followed a Mediterranean diet showed significant improvement in sleep quality, particularly for those aged 65 to 75.

"Above this balanced diet pattern was correlated negatively with the following: sleep and sleep disruption and sleep adequacy issues," says Mary Yannakoulia, Senior Author, Ph.D., Department of Nutrition and Diet, Harokopio University, Greece.

"Interestingly, we have also stated that sleep time (number of hours of sleep) is not significantly related to the Mediterranean diet," she said. Sleep quality is generally seen as a more comprehensive index, making it the key sleep metric for dietary decisions, while the length of sleep tends to be less vulnerable and not substantially correlated with diet.

Dr. Yannakoulia and her team claim many factors will play a part in enhancing the sleep quality of this specific anti-inflammatory eating pattern.

Mind Diet is Sound Sleep Encouraged

"The low sleep quality is related to elevated inflammatory and oxidation markers. Anti-inflammatory factors and antioxidant properties are commonly attributed to the Mediterranean dietary pattern," says Dr. Yannakoulia4-6.

You may be able to sleep at half noon and wake up at seven o'clock, but if your sleep is constantly disturbed, the amount is not important because the quality is very inadequate.

As inflammation may lead to sleep disruptions, they proposed that the rates of inflammation would decrease by adopting an anti-inflammatory diet – an approach that included fruit, vegetables, nuts, fish, olive, and whole grains; or a Mediterranean diet.

"The ties between Mediterranean diets and sleep quality could be explained by vascular pathways, as are good sources of melatonin, a neurohormone which modulates circadian rhythms and, inter alia, is involved in the slap-wake cycle via promotion of sleep and subsequence, among other factors."

Avoiding Inflammation Key to Reducing Chronic Diseases

It is important to note that, in addition to sleep, anti-inflammatory foods such as those containing the Mediterranean diet have a reduced risk of dying, including heart disease, certain cancers, and diabetes, as highlighted by another recent study.

Swedish scientists estimate that eating anti-inflammatory foods like fruits and vegetables, tea and coffee, single-saturated fats (e.g., olive and canola oils) nuts and avoiding pro-inflammatory meals — red food, fried meats, chips, and soda — reduce by 20%, cardiovascular disease and 13%, all causes of death.

A review of recent research investigating the relationship between different diets and disease potential published in the British Medical Journal further indicates the importance of adopting a diet based around anti-inflammatory food of the Mediterranean type. The literature review concludes that dietary patterns are closely related to disease prevention rather than individual foods.

No Matter Your Age, a mind Diet Is Beneficial

"The best way to sleep and improve your health is to balance the foods you chose to eat with those you have avoided," says Dr. Yannakoulia. If you wish to improve your sleep and reduce your risk of chronic disease in the near future, commit yourself to a healthy food pattern, which constructs meals around anti-inflammatory foods and sets free of fried, fast, and processed foods.

Dr. Fung emphasizes that while the anti-inflammatory aspects of the Mediterranean diet are significant, these foods also have other advantages. Adiponectin, a hormone responsible for regulating glucose levels, and facilitating fatty-acid breakdown, can increase the Mediterranean diet, which is important for healthy sleeping cycles, as well as to reduce the risk of diabetes, obesity, heart disease and possibly arthritis and osteoporosis, besides the anti-inflammatory and anti-oxidative effects.

If you are stuck in a cycle of too little sleep, too little food, too little exercise, and stress, a good starting point is to adjust your diet. The body can produce more of a hormone called ghrelin without sufficient sleep, and now send a signal to the brain that you need to feed. Sleep deficiency often reduces leptin, the hormone that causes the brain to slow feeding.

On the other hand, too little leptin tells the brain that more food is needed. By taking a Mediterranean diet-based approach, you are likely to sleep healthier, control your digestive hormone and, most importantly, reduce the overall risk of chronic diseases, which would otherwise worsen with age.

Moving Toward a Plant-based Approach is Key to Long-Term Health

Dr. Fung tells EndocrineWeb that while the Mediterranean diet represents a balanced eating strategy, the most important aim is to find the exact food plan, the one that fits best for you, and which can (more or less) be held every day.

Also, if you do not have to stick to a Mediterranean diet strictly, Dr. Fung suggests moving towards a more plant-based diet that includes: 'fruit, vegetables, whole grains, herbal proteins (e.g., beans, seeds, and nuts) and fish.'

While eating habits can encourage health over a lifetime, there are some foods everyone needs. For starters, it is important to get some green leafy vegetables every day; you have to choose the kinds of greens (e.g., kale, spinach, chard Swiss, Watercress, Roman, Boston, Bibb, etc.).

She also stresses the importance of gut microbes and recommends that you have low-fat, unsweetened yogurt daily in your diet. [Tip: add fresh or frozen fruit and nuts for delicious and good anti-inflammatory boost].

What about additions? Dr. Fung answers, "High-quality research has consistently shown that [nutritional] supplements benefit little in a well-nourished population," in other words, obtain the nutrients that are necessary from foods that you eat.

Sleep along with a balanced diet, daily exercise, and an effort to maintain low stress are important elements for healthier lives at any age and are the best path forward if you are graciously committed to aging.

While the Sleep in Aging research centered on an elderly population, the results indicate that the Mediterranean diet will have an equivalent impact on the patterns of sleep in young adults, Dr. Yannakoulia says.

Cardiovascular Disease

The MIND diet encourages eating high-fiber, complex carbs, vitamins, minerals, healthy fats, and phytochemicals in plant-based foods. MIND dietary nutrients decreased heart disease levels, heart disease death, total cholesterol, and HDL cholesterol relative to lower-fat diets, based on observational and clinical research meta-analysis.

The use of pure olive oil, the primary fat in the MIND diet, helps to reduce heart failure, plaque build-up in the lungs, unregular heartbeat, and heart disease.

The abundance of flavonoids in berries has been correlated with lower LDL cholesterol, triglycerides, lower blood pressure, and overall better heart safety (clinical, observatory, and animal studies).

Diabetes

Compared to low-fat diets, consuming high amounts of whole grains, fruit and vegetables strengthened the regulation of blood sugar and reduced the overall incidence of type 2 diabetes by about 20 percent

In a study of over 400 observational studies, the relationship between the major food groups in the MIND (all grains, vegetables, nuts, legumes, and fish) and type 2 diabetes were examined. You found that:

Reducing intake of "high-risk" foods (rough and refined meats, sugar beverages) has tripled the incidence of type 2 diabetes;

The incidence of type 2 diabetes was 42 percent decreased by the intake of sufficient amount of whole grains (2 servings per day), fruit (2-3 portions/day) and vegetables (2-3 portions/day)

Consumption of 50g / day of whole grains alone reduced type 2 diabetes by 25%

For another study, the majority of MIND diets were correlated with a decrease in the prevalence of type 2 diabetes of 20% (18 observational studies).

WEIGHT LOSS

The MIND diet is designed for brain health, although the focus on the whole, herbal food and the reduction of sweets, milk, fried and fast foods can encourage healthy loss of weight. The diet is also rich in carbohydrates and low in high calories foods.

Plant-based food (legumes and whole grains) reduced weight gain and obesity in observational and clinical trials better than high-protein, low-fat, and low-glycemic-index diets.

A cluster of disorders that raise the risk of obesity is metabolic syndrome. In the retrospective sample of nearly 800 young adults, olive oil, fruits, whole grains, legumes, and nuts lowered the risk of metabolic syndrome by 35% and decreased weight gain.

DEPRESSION

MIND diets, high in plant-based foodstuffs, reduced in several studies (clinical and observational) the rate of depression. The protective effects are possibly caused by the intake of a mixture of these foods rather than individual nutrients.

The DASH Diet (one of the parent diets of the MIND diet) improved mood and decreased symptoms of depression during a clinical study of 95 postmenopausal women for 14 weeks.

In an observational study of almost 16,000 adults, a decreased incidence of depression was associated with sticking to the Mediterranean diet for ten years. Such findings are attributed to foods that are also present in the MIND diet (vegetables, legumes, whole grains, nuts, fish).

Parkinson's Disease

Diäts that are rich in Mediterranean foods and MIND diets reduced the incidence of Parkinson's disease by 13 percent in observational studies of over 1.5 million people.

The MIND diet slowed down the progression of Parkinson's disease symptoms such as tremor and impaired coordination in another study of more than 700 older people.

The MIND Diet May Reduce Harmful Beta-Amyloid Proteins

Researchers are also of the belief that the MIND diet will help the brain minimize potentially harmful beta-amyloid protein.

Beta-amyloid proteins are normal protein fragments in the body. They can, however, accumulate and form brain plaques, disrupting contact between brain cells and eventually contributing to brain cell death.

Many scientists believe that these plaques are one of the main causes of Alzheimer's disease.

Animal and test-tube studies indicate that antioxidants and vitamins contained in many MIND diets can help prevent beta-amyloid plaques from forming in the brain.

Besides, the MIND diet reduces saturated fats and trans fats in foods that have been shown to raise beta-amyloid protein levels in the brains of mice.

Human evaluation studies have found a double chance of Alzheimer's disease correlated with the intake of these fats. It is important to remember, however, that such work can not prove cause and effect. Regulated, higher-quality studies are required to find out exactly how the MIND diet can support brain health.

Researchers conclude that MIND foods contain nutrients that can help prevent the development of beta-amyloid plaque, a possible cause of Alzheimer's disease.

MIND DIET SHOPPING LIST

The diet, which is low in added sugar and saturated fat, emphasizes omega-3 fatty acids, beans, legumes, fruits, or whole grain, as well as small quantities of olive oil.

The MIND diet – a Mediterranean and DASH hybrid – which also emphasizes fruits and leafy greens- is promising as a means to reduce the risk of Alzheimer's disease specifically. It is important to combine dietary efforts with regular exercise, socialization, and intellectual pursuit of a total brain support strategy.

Here are some foods to put in your cart on your next journey to the grocery store:

Fish

Fish: salmon, herring, mackerel, and tuna (those are the best in omega-3s.) Aim to serve 4-ounces, two or three days a week.

Nuts and seeds

Flaxseed or flax meal (watch amounts of stools greater than two cubic centimeters a day).

Walnuts

Brazilian nuts, filberts, almonds, peanuts, sunflowers, sesame seeds (raw or roasted, ideally not salted). Keep portions with a 1/8 cup serving at least 1/4 cup/day for calorie regulation. (Watch portions.)

Non-hydrogenated nut butter: Look for natural salt-free options, including peanut butter, almond butter, and tahini.

Vegetables

Greens leafy: spinach, kale, swiss chard, cod, mixed greens.

New and frozen vegetables, potatoes, onions, and tomatoes (rich in lutein), peppers, carotenoids, etc.

Legumes

Lentils, chickpeas, white and black beans (If you buy canned beans, look for lower varieties of salt or at least rinse beans underwater before serving.)

Fruits

Blueberries (may help to prevent oxidative stress in the brain).

Many fresh, frozen, and unsweetened canned and dried fruit (Citrus included an apple daily).

Pomegranate or juice (If juice, limit to 2 oz./day. Dilute with ice or water).

Whole grains

Oats, whole wheat, kamut, rye, farro, millet, quinoa, brown rice

Good Fats

- Avocado

- Olive oil

Beverages

Coffee (1-2 cups/day) can help focus; can prevent moderated neurogenerative diseases.

Teabags black or green (Try 2-3 cups/day hot or iced) to create freshly flavored tea. Containing caffeine and catechins that are flavonoid and antioxidant battles.

Treat

Dark chocolate (1/2-1 ounce a day offers all the benefits, including antioxidative, stimulants, and mood-enhancing endorphins.

Spices

Turmeric (contains anti-inflammatory properties)

Oregano, other fresh herbs.

MEAL PLAN SAMPLE FOR SEVEN DAYS

It does not have to be difficult to make meals for the MIND diet. Focus your meals around the ten foods and dietary groups that are recommended to stay away from the five foods that have to be restricted.

Here is a meal plan for seven days to get you started:

Monday

Breakfast: Overnight oats with strawberries.

Lunch: Burrito bowl with brown rice, black beans, fajita vegetables, grilled chicken, salsa, and guacamole.

Dinner: Mediterranean salad with olive-oil-based dressing, grilled chicken, whole-wheat pita.

Tuesday

Breakfast: Wheat toast with avocado, omelet with peppers and onions.

Lunch: Grilled salmon, side salad with olive-oil-based dressing, brown rice.

Dinner: Grilled chicken sandwich, blackberries, and carrots.

Wednesday

Breakfast: Greek yogurt with peanut butter and banana.

Lunch: Chicken and vegetable stir-fry, brown rice.

Dinner: Mexican-style salad with mixed greens, black beans, red onion, corn, grilled chicken, and olive-oil-based dressing.

Thursday

Breakfast: Steel-cut oatmeal with strawberries, hard-boiled eggs.

Lunch: Whole-wheat spaghetti with turkey meatballs and marinara sauce, side salad with olive-oil-based dressing.

Dinner: Baked trout, collard greens, black-eyed peas.

Friday

Breakfast: Wheat toast with almond butter, scrambled eggs.

Lunch: Greek-seasoned baked chicken, oven-roasted potatoes, side salad, wheat lunch roll.

Dinner: Chili made with ground turkey.

Saturday

Breakfast: Greek yogurt with raspberries, topped with sliced almonds.

Lunch: Chicken gyro on whole-wheat pita, cucumber, and tomato salad.

Dinner: Fish tacos on whole wheat tortillas, brown rice, pinto beans.

Sunday

Breakfast: Spinach frittata, sliced apple, and peanut butter.

Lunch: Curry chicken, brown rice, lentils.

Dinner: Tuna salad sandwich on wheat bread, plus carrots and celery with hummus.

After every meal, you should drink a glass of wine to meet the MIND diet guidelines. Nuts will make a large snack, too.

Most salad dressings in the shop are not primarily made of olive oil, but your own salad dressings can be made easily at home.

Combine three parts extra virgin olive oil with one part of balsamic vinegar to make a simple balsamic vinaigrette. Add some Dijon mustard, salt, and pepper and blend well. Mix well.

MIND diet meal planning is quick and fast. Focus your meals on the ten encouraging foods and try not to use the five foods that need to be limited.

MIND DIET RECIPES

BREAKFAST RECIPES

Begin your day with a brain-building cereal breakfast such as steel-cut oats, which contains nuts and berries. In particular, Schwartz claims that blueberry promotes neural safety as it is filled with an antioxidant known as anthocyanin. All kinds of antioxidants found in berries and other plant foods combat oxidative harm. "The evidence indicates that Alzheimer's disease the cognitive impairment has to do with oxidative stress," Schwartz says. Their combination of unsaturated fats and fiber is unsaturated for the health of the brain. And whole grains, Schwartz says, 'are linked to lower blood pressure and blood sugar control,' which are both essential for the proper functioning of the brain.

Oatmeal and scrambled egs are two great breakfasts for this diet. Oatmeal is a whole grain, and eggs are a neutral material that can be used to hold together a whole lot of MIND food ingredients.

Oatmeal

Simple oatmeal is typically bland. 1/4 cup of fast cooking oatmeal plus 1/2 cup of water and maybe some salt. Cook over low heat in a cup, stirring from time to time so that it does not stick to the rim. Cook until sticky.

Or you can throw it into the oven, just do so in a high side bowl, so it doesn't boil over. The cooking time depends on the power of the microwave and whether you want runny, smooth, or something between them. It normally takes 1 to 3 minutes. First, cook for one minute, then stir, then for another minute, then stir and start until the time it takes for your perfect oatmeal is reached. Cook for half the time, stir and then put the remainder of the time in the microwave and cook again, stir again, and have your oatmeal.

And the taste is... amazing. The MIND diet is not lawful for brown sugar and cream — and a step down the road to brain fog. Not unexpectedly, many people don't like oatmeal. Instead of water, cooking with brown rice milk or almond milk greatly enhances the taste.

Adding fruits and nuts during cooking enhances it. Sprinkle a little stevia on top, pour over it some brown rice milk or almond milk, and have a wonderful meal.

Other types:

    • Use different forms of oats: standard oats, steel-cut oats, scotch oats, oats.

    • Use additional grains: wheat cream, polenta, couscous, quinoa.

• Change the form of berries and use them on top fresh rather than fried.

• Using different types of nuts on top rather than cooked oatmeal.

• Before cooking, add dried blueberries or dried cranberries.

• Add 1 tsp of almond meal and mix before cooking.

Overnight oats

INGREDIENTS:

- 1 8 ounces mason jar.

- ½ cup rolled oats.

- ½ to 1 cup of almond milk.

- ¼ to 1 tsp vanilla.

- ½ cup berries (blueberries and strawberries work well).

How to:

Put all the ingredients in a jar and Stir. Place lid on the jar and refrigerate overnight.

Chocolate Overnight Oats w/ Strawberry Vanilla Sauce

The ultimate balanced breakfast dessert is these Chocolate Overnight Oats with Chia Seeds & Moist Strawberry Vanilla Sauce {gluten-free, vegan}!

INGREDIENTS:

- 1 tablespoon chia seeds.

- One teaspoon pure vanilla extract.

- 1 cup strawberries frozen & thawed or fresh.

- 1/3 cup gluten-free oats.

- One teaspoon pure maple syrup.

- 1/2 cup non-dairy milk of choice.

- 1 pinch salt.

- Cacao Nibs optional, for serving.

- 1/8 teaspoon salt.

- 5-ounce Chocolate Coconut Yogurt.

How to:

In a glass jar or bowl, place oats, yogurt, milk, chia seeds, and salt. Live overnight in the refrigerator or for 3-4 hours until the oats are softened. Place them in the fridge too if frozen strawberries are used, allow them to thaw overnight, or freeze them in the microwave before making the compound.

Keep the Vanilla Sauce Hot Strawberry

Steam a medium fire saucepan. Stir in thawed strawberries, then sprinkle with a gourd or potato mash for about 1 minute. Add maple syrup and vanilla and cook for 1-2 minutes additional.

Serving.

Take strawberry compote over the overnight oats and sprinkle cacao nibs over it if desired.

NOTES:

You can make several jars of oats in advance, and keep them well covered in the fridge for up to 3 days before serving. You can also cook the strawberry compote in advance, lock it in the refrigerator and heat it before serving in the microwave.

Make Low FODMAP: coconut yogurt is low FODMAP per Monash app (2/8/20), but read marks as ingredients may alter. Lactose-free yogurt (i.e., Green Valley or Siggi's) + cocoa powder can also be used as an alternative to chocolate milk yogurt.

Egg dishes

Eggs are neutral to the MIND diet but a perfect vegetable carrier. Depending on their preparation, a simple combination of eggs, chopped vegetables, with or without a small cheese, becomes many egg dishes.

Scrambles

A scramble is eggs scrambled with sliced vegetables. Ideally, you 're only going to have a lot of veggies with eggs.

INGREDIENTS:

- ½ cup young spinach.

- ¼ cup chopped onions.

- Two eggs scrambled.

- Olive oil.

- ¼ cup sliced mushrooms.

How to:

Place just enough olive oil in the pan to prevent vegetables from sticking. Remove onions and mushrooms, fry over low heat, stirring, until the onions are slightly translucent and mushrooms just beginning to turn green. Add spinach, stir before just beginning to wilt. Remove eggs and whisk to mix. Scrape them together as they start to cook. When eggs are fully good, flip the whole thing. Cook to desired moistness/dryness.

Frittata

INGREDIENTS:

- ½ cup young spinach.

- Three eggs scrambled.

- ¼ cup sliced mushrooms.

- ½ to 1-ounce grated cheese.

- ¼ cup chopped onions.

How to:

Start with one more egg in the same way as the scramble:

Preheat the oven to 350 ° C.

Oil or grind 3 cups of muffin or cupcakes

Pour ample olive oil into the pot to avoid sticking vegetables. Add onions and mushrooms, fry over low heat, and stir until the onions are slightly translucent and mushrooms begin to change color. Apply spinach, stir until it wakes. Connect the eggs and blend.

Put into the three muffin tins and divided evenly.

Sprinkle the cheese, split evenly.

Bake for 15 to 20 minutes, slightly melted eggs and cheese.

Quiche

INGREDIENTS:

- ¼ cup grated cheese.

- ½ cup sliced mushrooms.

- Four eggs scrambled.

- ½ cup chopped onions.

- 1 cup fresh spinach.

How to:

Preheat the oven to 350 ° C. Fill a 9-inch pie pot olive oil.

Pour ample olive oil into the pot to avoid sticking vegetables. Add onions and mushrooms, fry over low heat, and stir until the onions are slightly translucent and mushrooms begin to change color. Apply spinach, stir until it wakes. Connect the eggs and blend. Remove the cheese and blend it.

Put in the saucepan.

Bake for 1/2 hour at 350 or until the toothpick inserted is dry.

Omelet

INGREDIENTS:

- Two eggs scrambled.

- ¼ cup chopped onions.

- ½ cup young spinach.

- Olive oil.

- ¼ cup sliced mushrooms.

How to:

In a little olive oil, cook the vegetables. Hold warm on low heat.

Place the eggs in a bowl or omelet.

Cook over low heat until the eggs are set in the pancake shape. Flip and cook until the eggs are done a little longer. Pile the veggies on top, fold the "pancake" over and inside the veggies.

Apply two tablespoons grated cheese before folding the pancakes or sprinkle the 2 tbsp on top of the omelet if you prefer cheese in the omelet.

Green Eggs, No Ham {Kale Pesto with Scrambled Eggs and Cherry Tomatoes}

INGREDIENTS:

- One tablespoon extra-virgin olive oil.

- Four eggs.

- 1 cup cherry tomatoes sliced in half.

- 1/2 cup fresh basil packed.

- 1/2 to 1 clove garlic or to taste.

- Salt and fresh ground black pepper to taste.

- Vegetable oil or butter for frying eggs.

- Two tablespoons pine nuts.

- 2 cups chopped kale well packed.

How to:

Prepare the kale pesto: put in the food processor kale, basil, pine nuts, olive oil, and garlic and combine pulse. Season to taste with salt and pepper and reserve.

Fry the pot with vegetable oil or butter and scrap the eggs in medium sun.

Divide the eggs into two portions and finish with half the kale pesto mixture and half the cherry tomatoes, each serving.

NOTE:

Nutrition Notes: Gluten-free and vegetarian, of course. Consider serving a vegan choice with scrambled tofu.

Easy Gluten-Free Berry Crisp

INGREDIENTS:

- 1/4 cup brown sugar.

- 1/4 cup sorghum flour or brown rice flour.

- One tablespoon maple syrup optional though.

- 2 cups blueberries.

- Two tablespoons chia seeds.

- 1/2 cup gluten-free oats.

- 1/4 cup tapioca starch.

- 1/4 cup virgin coconut oil melted, plus extra for ramekins.

- Juice from 1/2 Meyer lemon.

- 2 cups sliced strawberries.

- 1/8 teaspoon salt.

How to:

Preheat oven to 350 ° C. In a mixing bowl, add strawberries, blueberries, lemon juice, and chia seeds.

Add oats, flours, brown sugar, coconut oil, and salt together in another cup.

Grease 4 ramekins with cocoa oil, then spoon fruit mix into ramekins and combine oatmeal/flour. Place about 20 minutes on a baking sheet or until it is crispy.

Remove slightly from the oven to cool, then serve.

NOTE:

Besides being vegan and gluten-free. This crisp berry oatmeal is also ideal for a low FODMAP diet. Feel free to substitute sorghum flour for another gluten-free grain, such as brown rice, millet, or quinoa.

Hazelnut-Crusted Halibut with Beet and Spinach Salad

The MIND diet suggests that you eat at least five days a week an ounce of nuts. One way to fill it is to strip the panko and cover fish (or chicken) with finely cut nuts. Here we were using hazelnuts, but almonds would fit just as well.

INGREDIENTS:

- 5 ounces fresh baby spinach.

- Three medium-sized navel oranges.

- Three large egg whites, beaten well.

- 3/4 cup finely chopped blanched hazelnuts.

- 1 1/4 teaspoon kosher salt, divided.

- Three tablespoons avocado oil or olive oil, divided.

- 1 1/2 tablespoon balsamic vinegar.

- 1 pkg. Precooked ready-to-eat beets, cut into wedges.

- Four skinless halibut fillets.

- 1/2 cup whole-wheat pastry flour.

- 3/4 teaspoon black pepper, divided.

How to:

In a shallow dish, put a meal. In a second shallow dish, placed white eggs. In a third shallow bowl, put the hazelnuts. Sprinkle fillets with 3⁄4 salt teaspoon and 1⁄2 pepper teaspoon. Dredge in flour and shake off the excess of 1 fillet at a time. Sprinkle in egg whites, then brush in hazelnuts and press to stick.

Heat 2 tablespoons of oil over medium in a big, non-stick skillet. Add fillets and cook until the nuts are slightly toasted, and the fillets are easy to flake 4 to 5 minutes a day with a fork. Move to board. Switch to board.

Cut the peel and the pith away from the orange flesh with a paring knife. Cut oranges, holding the fruit over a bowl for juices. Reserve segments (about 1 1⁄2 cups). Reserve segments. Add one tablespoon of vinegar, 1⁄2 tea cubicles of salt, 1/2 tea cubicle of pepper to cup, whisk to blend. Add the beets and spinach to the bowl. Divide salad and filets equally into four plates; cover with orange segments and drizzle with the remaining bowl vinaigrette.

Whole-Grain Pasta Primavera

Crisp-tender green veggies compliment chewy whole-grain pasta; they have some olive oil, flavors of red pepper, and feta. While this dish is delicious without the cheese, the recipe is genuinely sung by this bit of creaminess.

INGREDIENTS:

- 8 ounces uncooked whole-wheat penne.

- 4 cups broccoli florets (8 oz).

- 12 ounces asparagus, trimmed and cut into 2-inch pieces (about 2 cups).

- 1/2 cup fresh or frozen green peas.

- 1/4 cup olive oil.

- 1 teaspoon kosher salt.

- 1/4 teaspoon crushed red pepper flakes.

- 2 ounces crumbled feta cheese (about ½ cup), divided (optional) 3/4 cup torn basil leaves, divided.

How to:

Carry a big pot of water over high to a boil. Cook pasta 7 minutes. Add pasta. Fill in broccoli; cook for 2 minutes. Add asparagus and peas; cook for 2 minutes, if healthy. (If you use frozen peas, add the asparagus cooker into the pot, 2 minutes, and immediately remove it from the heat).

Return pasta and reserved cooking water to a low bowl. Add olive oil, salt, red pepper, 1/4 cup of feta, and 1/2 cup of basil. Cook, stirring gently, about 2 minutes until sauce thickens. Split pasta evenly between 4 bowls and top with 1/4 cup of feta and 1/2 cup of basil remaining.

Low-Carb Portabella Mushroom Baked Eggs

These portabella mushroom baked eggs are a simple and fast way to add a portion of your daily intake. You only need two ingredients for this breakfast and 20 minutes. Serve for a balanced meal with a slice of full grain toast and fruit. You can also add a side of sautéed kale or spinach to start your day with even more vegetable goodness.

INGREDIENTS:

- Olive oil cooking spray.

- Two portabella mushroom caps.

- Two large eggs.

How to:

400F heat oven. Line a parchment bakery or silicone baking sheet. Mist the lined bakery sheet with the mist.

Remove all other stems from the caps of the mushroom. Place each cap on the baker 's bottom faces up. Five minutes cooked. Cooked. Oven removes. Remove from the oven.

Crack one egg carefully into each mushroom shell. Return to the oven and bake for another 10-15 minutes, or until white and yolk are strong.

Remove and serve from the oven.

Baked Sweet Potato Noodles in Spicy Tomato Marinara

Vegetable noodles are full of brain-healthy phytonutrients, fiber, vitamins, and mineral products, also known as "voodles." You will use sweet potato noodles in this dish. Such tubers are loaded with vitamin C and vitamin A (or beta-carotene), which are antioxidants and helps to boost brain health.

In this dish, you'll get a healthy dose of B-vitamin, folate, sweet potatoes, and tomato sauce. Folate has demonstrated strong protection against cognitive health and dementia. Lycopene is also a major antioxidant in the tomato sauce.

INGREDIENTS:

- One medium sweet potato, peeled, washed and cut into 2 or 3 pieces.

- One tablespoon extra-virgin olive oil.

- One clove fresh garlic, minced.

- 1-15 ounce can pureed tomatoes.

- 1 teaspoon dried oregano.

- 1 teaspoon cinnamon.

- One teaspoon red pepper flakes.

- Dash of salt and black pepper.

- 1/8 cup fresh Parmesan cheese, grated.

How to:

Preheat 350F oven. Spiral each piece of sweet potato and placed it sideways in a bowl.

Add olive oil and garlic on the stovetop over medium heat; heat for a minute. Pour in the tomatoes pureed. Remove and add oregano, cinnamon, flakes of red pepper, salt, and pepper. Remove well and heat through.

Pour the marinara and mix until well-coated over sweet potato spirals. Spoon into an oven-safe dish and cook for 30-45 minutes or until softly cooked potatoes.

Oven removes. Remove from the oven. Sprinkle with cheese and immediately serve.

Sweet Potato Brussels Sprout Breakfast Hash

Looking for a nice weekend with a healthier breakfast than bacon and pancakes? This sweet potato hash breakfast is a good, healthy way to start your day. It is loaded with vegetables, so you get a dose of fiber first in the morning, and there are only eight ingredients there. Just roast some vegetables in the oven, crack some eggs and have a tasty, delicious breakfast or brunch.

INGREDIENTS:

- One small sweet potato, diced.

- 1/2 medium onion, diced.

- 1 1/2 cups brussels sprouts, halved.

- 1 tablespoon avocado oil.

- 1/2 teaspoon freshly ground black pepper.

- One tablespoon pure maple syrup.

- 1/4 tsp crushed red pepper flakes.

- Four large eggs.

How to:

425F hot oven. Place a 10-inch cast-iron pot in a preheated oven. After the pot has been heated, add oil and swirl around the bowl. Remove carrots, cabbage, Brussels, and black pepper. Remove to cover with oil. Bake for about 25-30 minutes, stirring about 10 minutes.

Remove the skillet and add maple syrup and red pepper. Remove from the oven.

Make four small egg holes.

Crack one egg carefully into each hole. Place your skillet back in the oven and cook for a further 5-10 minutes, as you like the center of your eggs.

Remove from the oven and eat as soon as possible.

Wild Blueberry Holiday Breakfast Crumble

This moist and easy breakfast is crowded. It includes wild blueberries, wholesome grain oats, healthy olive oil, and warm holiday spices such as cinnamon and mustard. When you try it and see how easy it is to produce, swap fruits in various seasons and play the topping too.

INGREDIENTS:

For the topping:

- ½ cup organic rolled oats.

- ½ cup Bob's Red Mill whole wheat pastry flour.

- ¼ cup Swerve granulated "sugar."

- ¼ cup almond slivers.

- ¼ cup raw pistachios, coarsely chopped.

- One tablespoon unsweetened organic coconut chips.

- 1 teaspoon cinnamon.

- ½ teaspoon cardamom.

- ¼ teaspoon nutmeg.

- Generous pinch of salt.

- ¼ cup olive oil.

For the filling:

- One 16-oz bag of frozen wild blueberries (about 3.5 cups)

- 2 oz dried mission figs (about ⅓ cup lightly packed, or 10-12 small and medium figs), coarsely chopped.

- One tablespoon arrowroot powder.

- One lemon, zest from the whole lemon, the juice from half the lemon.

- 1 tsp Watkins baking vanilla extract.

- ¼ cup balsamic vinegar.

- Pinch of salt.

How to:

Preheat to 350F. Preheat oven.

Make the top. Combine all ingredients except the olive oil in a medium bowl. Remove until uniformly combined. Add olive oil and blend until moisturized.

Make full. Mix blueberries, figs, arrowroot powder, citrus zest, lemon juice, vanilla extract, salt, and balsamic vinegar in another medium mixing bowl. Mix well together. Stir well.

Grate a 9-inch bakery with olive oil or butter slightly. Add filling. Add filling. Apply icing over the filling uniformly.

Cook 30 minutes. Bake 30 minutes. The fruit should be bubbling and browning. If not, give another five minutes to cook and re-check. Remove from oven and require 10 minutes of rest before serving.

It's all tasty on its own, but with a side of yogurt like Siggi 's new lactose-free yogurt, it's just as good.

Korean Danhobak (kabocha squash) Porridge

In the Korean language, this dish is called "hobakjuk" and can refer technically to turkey or squash porridge in winter. However, it is most commonly referred to as a squash called Danhobak (it is also known as kabocha squash). Short grain brown rice is a natural way of enhancing its silky, creamy texture.

This gentle, soothing porridge celebrates the subtle sweetness of kabocha squash naturally found.

INGREDIENTS:

For the Porridge:

- ½ cup sweet brown rice.

- One medium kabocha squash, about 4 lbs measured whole.

- 6 cups of water, ½ cup of water.

- Salt to taste.

- garnishes: red date, sliced; pine nuts, roasted sesame seeds.

- Optional: honey.

For the Mochi:

- ½ cup sweet rice flour.

- Five tablespoons of water.

How to:

Rinse and drain brown rice 3 to 5 times in cool water. Soak rice for at least 1 hour in clean water (can be achieved a day ahead).

Preheat the oven to 400F, 15 minutes, approximately.

In the meantime, the squash softened. Wash squash well, pierce with a fork or knife many times, and put in a large microwave-safe 3-inch dish. Four minutes of cooking time. Flip over the squash and cook 4 minutes longer. Let squash rest until cool enough, then cut into 2-4 pieces and toss it with neutral oil and then cut it off and roast for 20 minutes on the side of a flaked baking sheet. Remove skin until cool enough to treat. It's six to eight cups.

Keep the thickening fluid when squash is roasting. Drain soaked rice and add 1/2 cup of water to the blender. Mix well until liquified, and reserve until ready to use. Rinse out the blender easily.

Mix the squash in plenty, adding 6 cups of water slowly, until smooth. Shift mixed squash into a broad pot and heat to a low point.

Attach the brown rice-water mixture slowly and allow it to simmer for 10-15 minutes. Take salt and heat to compare.

Meanwhile, make dumplings for the rice cake. Start to boil a medium pot of water and make a big bowl of ice.

Heat 5 tablespoons of water, for example, in microwave oven or tea kettle.

In a medium bowl, put rice flour and slowly add hot water to cool enough to handle and then knead the dough for a few minutes.

Cut out a 1/2 teaspoon and roll the dough between the palms to make small balls (about 30 of them).

Fall 1-2 minutes into boiling water before you float.

Remove rice cake pimples and put them in the cold-water bath before they are ready to use.

Cover the top.

Pour soup into bowls, add a couple of rice cake dumplings and garnish. Drizzle with sweetheart if used. Live. Enjoy.

Strawberry and Pineapple Plate with Whiskey-Ginger Drizzle

Twice a week, the MIND diet calls for berries. Here's an easy snack created by a fantastic snack. Personally, with or without the drizzle, I would happily eat that, but it does add something really special and unexpected.

INGREDIENTS:

- ¼ cup whiskey.

- ½ tsp extra-virgin olive oil.

- ¼ tsp vanilla extract.

- 1 tsp freshly shredded ginger.

- 1 tbsp pineapple juice.

- ¼ cup pineapple slices.

- Eight strawberries.

- Optional garnishes: pink Himalayan salt, mint.

How to:

Combine a pinch of salt, whisky, olive oil, vanilla, ginger, and pineapple juice. Let rest for at least 10 minutes, but it's ideal for 30 minutes or more.

Arrange on a plate pineapple slices and strawberries and drizzle over liquid.

Garnish, if needed, with rose salt and mint leaves.

LUNCH RECIPES

Try a whole grain pasta with vegetables and grilled salmon for a fun lunch, says Schwartz, who recommends tossing greens like spinach, and fresh herbs when you prepare the pasta sauce. Not only have herbs and spices high antioxidant content, but they also make a good taste of food so that you can stick to your balanced diet much easier. Like fatty fish, salmon is filled with omega-3s, essential for brain memory functions.

For an additional boost to omega 3, eat a few walnuts as a snack in the afternoon. "Blood sugar stabilizes snacking between meals."

Sandwiches

Sandwiches are quite evident. Original: two full-grain bread pieces and inside a piece of meat or cheese.

Most sandwiches contain some type of mayonnaise, mustard, or ketchup spread over bread. It's easier to spray or brush on meat or cheese if you want to try olive oil, instead of attempting to spread it onto the plate, which can easily become soggy.

Additional vegetables include pickles (dill or sweet), tomatoes, and onion. The more vegetables you can add to the mind diet, the better.

Salads

Lettuce and dressing are a very simple salad. Boring. Boring. So, salad bars are so popular. And croutons do not follow the spirit of the MIND diet when contributing to crunch. Think of veggies, veggies, veggies, and an approach to the salad bar. Purchase one of these salad mixes, at least, with some carrots and add some tomatoes.

Basic salad bar:

Lettuce in any form or combination of salad, chalk, endive, baby spinach, or any other green leafy stuff. Try as many different salads as you can – a new favorite may be found.

Tomatoes – tomatoes or wedges of tomato or slices of tomato. Try the local farmer's market heritage tomatoes. Some are very sweet and very mild. Some of them have a slightly salty flavor. Some have a good love for tomatoes.

Veggies with dips go well in salads, too. Carrots, celery, broccoli, colic, peas, snow peas – all in the salads are fine.

To give the salad a little more body, you can add:

- Almonds (sliced).

- Chicken (shredded).

- Garbanzo beans.

- Kidney beans.

- Salmon.

- Shrimp (tiny salad size).

- Sunflower seeds.

- Tuna (light).

- Turkey (shredded).

- Walnuts (chopped).

Make the zillion veggie approach to your salad, and you've increased your salad 's nutrition many times. So long as you choose the right dressing of the salad.

It is shocking that sugar or, worse, high fructose corn syrup is included in the ingredients in many salad dressings. This is not in the MIND diet's spirit. When you drink from your lettuce, you have just moved it to the category 'sweets.'

Olive oil and vinegar of red wine instead create the traditional olive oil and vinegar. For 1 part of vinegar, using three parts of olive oil. That means three tbsp oil with one tbsp vinegar or 3/4 cup of vinegar with 1/4 cup. If you have to dress sweetly, add a little stevia.

Soups

When you make soup, I strongly advise you to make a bowl. You can also use a hot pot, but I find that these soups are less aromatic. Some herbal flavors get stronger, and you might have to adjust the seasoning if you have a favorite soup recipe for the crockpot.

If you don't want a crockpot, make the soup one day, so you can make sure that the liquid doesn't boil off, burning up the base ingredients. The other option is to put it in a jar covered in the oven and set it very low.

Soup is fluid that has long been cooked with something, whether in various combinations – vegetables, meat, poultry, fish, or seafood. If you put the vegetables in a little olive oil before you add the liquid, it tends to taste a bit better. If you add a little meat, it will also taste better if it is cooked before you add it to the soup. Spread it in olive oil as raw – like ground beef or ground Turkey, chop it as it is cooked, and then crumble into small pieces.

If you want vegetable soup with no meat, I strongly recommend the following Loaded Veggie Soup recipe. Different versions are available on the Web, and all taste good to me. It freezes well so that you can cook it once and eat it several times.

If you have a lot of meat, such as a pot roast or a lot of bones as your soup base, try the meat soup recipe after the Loaded Veggie.

Vegetable Soup

I hate vegetable canned soup. So, I was shocked when I tried the following Loaded Veggie Soup recipe. Very good! Very good! And it's good because for a month it's good enough to serve you and your neighbors.

INGREDIENTS:

- 2 – 3 Tbsp. olive oil.

- Four large carrots, cut in ½ to 1-inch chunks.

- 1/2 bunch of celery with leaves, chopped.

- Two medium-sized onions, chopped.

- Four large cloves of garlic, minced.

- 2 cups fresh mushrooms, sliced.

- 1 large green pepper.

- 1 large red pepper.

- One small head of broccoli, chopped.

- Four large vine-ripened tomatoes, chopped (can substitute canned diced tomatoes).

- 1 1/2 cups frozen corn.

- 1 1/2 cups fresh or frozen peas.

- 1 1/2 cups fresh or frozen green beans, cut into bite-sized pieces.

- Three red potatoes, scrubbed and cut into bite-sized pieces with skin on.

- One medium sweet potato, peeled and cut into bite-sized pieces.

- 1 1/2 cups brussels sprouts -if large, cut in half.

- 1/2 green cabbage, cut in bite-sized pieces (or use one bag coleslaw mix).

- 1 cup cauliflower, cut in bite-sized pieces.

- Two zucchini, cut into bite-sized pieces.

- One small head broccoli, cut into bite-sized pieces.

- 1 cup fresh spinach.

- 10 cups of liquid of choice: water, vegetable broth, chicken broth, or beef broth.

- 3 tbsp. tomato paste.

- Three large bay leaves.

- 2 tbsp. dried basil.

- 1 tbsp. thyme.

- 1 tsp. cumin.

- 1/2 tsp. black pepper.

How to:

Salt to drink. Salt to eat. (If you substitute a meat broth with wine, make sure you try before adding.)

In a large pot or skillet, add olive oil over medium heat and then add veggies one at a time, mixing and frying a little. Do not remove anything-just add and stir until everything is in your pot. Some people like chopping, adding and mixing, chopping, adding and mixing the next food. This helps, especially if you don't have much chopping space.

Attach your choice of the liquid, mix. Dip 1⁄4 cup of liquid and stir into the tomato paste until the paste dissolves and there are no lumps left and then return to the bowl. Remove to spread evenly, and then add all herbs and pepper. (I recommend leaving the salt out for a while). When cooking in a kettle, cook for 6 to 8 hours at low temperature. You can also make this in a Dutch oven or in a pot: simmer for 3 to 4 hours at low temperature.

If needed, savor and add salt or pepper or more tomato paste (or other favorite herbs or spices).

Return to room temperature once you have eaten as much as you can. Store one or two serving sizes in your chosen container in the freezer.

Veggie soup variations

If you like your soup a bit spicy, try adding crushed pepper flakes, jalapeno peppers, your favorite hot sauce, or anything you like in that line.

If you like meat in your soup, skip a pound of ground beef, ground chicken, or ground turkey before adding any liquid, then you're getting small pieces of crumble. Use meat and fruit juices. Remaining stew meat or pot roast can also be used, or chicken or turkey remaining cut into small pieces. Make sure you add any juices or gravy with remaining meat or poultry.

Increase or add any herbs you enjoy. Take something you don't like out. Leave it out. Okra, parsley and/or cilantro have some recipes. Interestingly, there is a gene that tastes like soap. If you are like me and you like cilantro, don't feel compelled to add it.

Another change:

When some veggies like carrots, maize, or spinach are barely cooked, leave them off until approximately 15 minutes before the end. Then add them. Add them.

Meat and poultry-based soups

Both meat and poultry add more flavor to a soup if first baked. The two most delicious methods are either to roast or to cook in a pot for 6 to 8 hours. Cut into pieces when you cook in a crockpot. Instead of covering with broth, simply add liquid to cover approximately half the meat. The taste of the juices is better. Cook the vegetables individually – only to get maximum taste and crispness for a short time.

INGREDIENTS:

- 1 to 3 pounds of roasted meat/poultry/bones, cooked, cut into bite-sized pieces, with juices/gravy.

- 1 tsp olive oil.

- 1 onion, diced.

- Four red potatoes, quartered.

- ½ pound mushrooms, sliced.

- ½ pound baby carrots.

- Two stalks celery, sliced into 1/4-inch slices.

- 4 cups meat or chicken broth.

- 1 bay leaf.

- ½ tsp thyme.

- ¼ tsp cumin.

- ½ tsp basil.

- ¼ tsp pepper.

How to:

If using ground beef, brush with the beef in the olive oil, cut and stir as it is cooking until it ends in small crumbs.

Add vegetables, cook, and combine until the onions are translucent.

Add all herbs and broth. Apply additional salt and pepper if desired, and taste.

If you prefer softer vegetables, cook the soup 1 to 2 hours before serving.

Meat soup types:

- Jumping veggies. Remove cooked meat and any available juices. Use a cup of broth to make gravy. Combine well and serve over noodles or rice.

- Add a little lower sweetness and thicken the broth after cooking the meat and veggies with two tbsp of flour per cup of liquid, then stew.

- Add additional vegetables, as many as you want.

Lentil, Arugula, and Avocado Salad

It blends two MIND force players — lentils and greens — and gets together in just 15 minutes. This salad is suitable for a weekend dinner. The messy, probiotic-packed yogurt dressing and avocado make it so easy to make a salad.

INGREDIENTS:

- 3/4 cup plain whole-milk Greek yogurt.

- Two tablespoons fresh lemon juice (from 1 lemon).

- 1 tablespoon honey.

- 3/4 teaspoon kosher salt.

- 1/2 teaspoon black pepper.

- 3 ounces baby arugula (3 cups).

- 3 cups thinly sliced radicchio (from 1 small head).

- 3 cups multicolored cherry tomatoes, halved (from 2 pints).

- 1/2 cup roasted pumpkin seeds (pepitas), divided.

- 1 (17.6-oz.) pkg. cooked lentils, rinsed and dried on paper towels.

- One avocado, cut into cubes.

How to:

In a medium cup, whisk milk, lemon juice, sugar, salt, and pepper together.

Place the pumpkin seeds in the bread bowl in arugula, radicchio, tomatoes, and 1⁄4 cup. Add 1⁄2 cup of yogurt and brush gently. Divide between 4 bowls. Top with sunglasses, avocados, and 1⁄4 cup of pumpkin seeds leftover. Remaining dressing drizzle.

Crunchy Lentil Tacos, avocado Feta Guacamole

INGREDIENTS:

- One tablespoon avocado oil or other high-oleic vegetable oil.

- 2 1/2 cups pre-cooked lentils (i.e. Trader Joe's Ready-to-Eat Steamed Lentils).

- One small sweet onion finely chopped and divided.

- 1 teaspoon ground cumin.

- 1 teaspoon chili powder.

- 1/4 teaspoon ground black pepper.

- 1/8 teaspoon salt or to taste.

- 1/4 cup water.

- Three small avocados or two medium to large avocados.

- 1 cup crumbled feta cheese.

- 8-12 crunchy taco shells.

- Optional for serving: Chopped lettuce, chopped tomato, cilantro, hot sauce.

How to:

Heat a large skillet over medium heat and add oil and 1/2 cup of chopped ointment to the saucepan. Stir until the onion is supplanted, about 2 minutes. Add cooked lentils and mix, add the cumin, chili powder, salt, pepper, and water to the lens/onion mix and mix well. Turn heat to low to sparkle during avocado feta guacamole preparation.

Retire the skin and pit from the avocados and placed them in a medium dish. Mash the avocados with a fork and then add the rest of chopped onion and feta and combine well.

Spoon meat lens mix into a serving bowl and place it on the table together with the taco shells, avocado feta guacamole, and the appropriate taco fittings so that everyone can use the 'Taco Bar Style' to themselves.

NOTES:

These crunchy lentil tacos packed with protein, fiber, and calcium are also a fabulous plant-based iron source which supplies 36% of your recommended daily intake in 3 tacos.

For a vegan choice, omit feta cheese.

The food supplied is for 2 or 3 tacos per meal, depending on how hungry you are. In reality, tacos are quite hungry, but have, by all means, if you're extra hungry.

Add a fresh fruit side, and you'll have a full meal!

Easy Lentil Salad with Lemon Vinaigrette

INGREDIENTS:

- 2 cups chopped kale.

- 3/4 cup cherry tomatoes sliced in half.

- 1/2 cup chopped Radicchio.

- 1/2 cup cooked lentils.

- Two tablespoons slivered almonds.

- One tablespoon extra-virgin olive oil.

- Juice from 1/4 of a lemon.

- Sea salt and black pepper to taste.

How to:

Kale, cherry tomatoes, Radicchio optional, lentils, and almonds in a bowl of salads. Add olive oil, citrus fruit juice, and salt and pepper to taste. Then toss thoroughly, then serve.

Salmon-Kale Summer Rolls

Shake the new and fun-to-eat omega-3-rich salmon, brown rice, and many sweet, crunchy veggies for supper. For a spicy, creamy kick, mix a dipping mayonnaise and sriracha sauce or simply add a drizzle of gluten-free tamari to those crowd pleasures.

INGREDIENTS:

- 1 cup uncooked brown sushi rice.

- Two teaspoons light brown sugar.

- 4 1/2 tablespoon rice vinegar, divided.

- 3/4 teaspoon kosher salt, divided.

- Five large Lacinato kale leaves stems removed, leaves very thinly sliced.

- 1 tablespoon canola oil.

- 8 round rice paper sheets.

- 1 1/2 very thinly sliced radishes (12 oz.).

- 1 1/2 cups very thinly sliced Persian or English cucumbers (about 7 oz.).

- One avocado, cut into 16 slices.

- 6 ounces thinly sliced smoked salmon.

How to:

In a strainer, put rice. Rinse under cold running water for about 1 minute until clear. Move rice to a tiny cup; add 1 1/2 cups of water. Cover and put over high to a boil. Reduce to medium-low heat and cook 40 minutes. Remove from heat and allow 20 minutes to stand. Transfer to a medium-sized bowl and toss with sugar, 3 1/2 vinegar tablespoon, and 1/2 salt teaspoon. Let it cool about 20 minutes.

Put kale in a bowl with olive oil and one tablespoon of vinegar and 1/4 teaspoon of salt. Massage vigorously with fingers for 1 to 2 minutes, until the leaves are tender.

Fill a large, shallow dish with warm water at a depth of 1 inch. Place one sheet of rice on the water; let stand only about 30 seconds until soft. Move to a smooth surface of the sheet. Arrange 1/8 of the radishes, 1/8 of the cucumbers, and two avocado pieces in a row across the wrapper center, leaving at every end a 1-inch margin. Finish with 1/4 cup of rice, pinch together grains as you seal. Add 1/4 cup of peanut and 3/4 ounce of salmon. Fold the ends of the sheet and roll up, jelly-roll mode. Push the seam gently to close. Place roll, seam side down, on a platter lined in a damp towel or paper, and cover with another damp towel of paper so that it is not dry. Repeat the rest of the ingredients cycle. Serve immediately.

Dreamy Turkey and Veggie English Muffin Sammie

This powerful Sammy is full for lunch on an entire grain of English muffin, with a lean, white turkey breast for a protein-packed bite. Combine this with a smear of creamy avocado for brain-healthy fats and potassium for control of blood pressure and fresh lime juice for extra citrus fruit and antioxidant flavored with vitamin C.

Add a few slices of radish for a clean, crunchy, and low-calorie root vegetable, which contributes to a medium-size calorie mere one calorie. It's no brainer! It's no brainer! Lay on top a Roman leaf, add more starch, dietary vitamin K, folate, and calcium for a hint.

INGREDIENTS:

- One whole-grain English muffin, halved and toasted.

- ¼ small ripe avocado.

- Freshly squeezed juice from half of a small lime.

- Salt and pepper to taste.

- One medium radish, thinly sliced.

- 3 ounces roasted turkey breast, sliced.

- ½ Romaine lettuce leaf.

How to:

Place your English muffin in a toaster or toaster oven. Toast for about 30 to 60 seconds, depending on how you like it toasted. Remove the plate and put it on.

Spread a pinch of salt and pepper and sprinkle on half of the muffin with the avocado, spritz with the lime juice. Cover with slices of radish.

Pile up the breast of turkey and lettuce. To complete the sandwich, place the other half of the muffin on top.

Chicken and Black Bean Cilantro Lime Burrito

Kick your brain health with this chicken burrito filled with veggie and white meat. The spread of avocado is filled with potassium, good unsaturated fats, and dietary fiber. It is also filled with vitamin C, an antioxidant that can improve your immunity and protect your cells drastically weakened.

The magnetic, shredded chicken-breast is flavored with anti-inflammatory spices — cayenne and smoked paprika — and the sprinkle of black beans provides rich amounts of dietary fiber and protein. Even the chopped roman lettuce, a green leaf packed of vitamins A, K, and potassium, contains brain-healthy omega-3 fats. Finally, add some additional cilantro leaves of vitamin K and potassium, then cut some red cherry tomatoes to a red burst and further amplify lycopene vitamin C, potassium, and antioxidants.

Each single ingredient in this safe chicken burrito recipe gives the body something good if you don't get the picture yet!

INGREDIENTS:

- One teaspoon cayenne pepper.

- One teaspoon smoked paprika.

- One teaspoon ground turmeric.

- 1 teaspoon kosher salt.

- 1 teaspoon black pepper.

- 2 to 4-ounce skinless chicken breasts.

- 1/2 cup apple cider vinegar.

- 1/8 cup water.

- One tablespoon low-sodium Worcestershire sauce.

- One tablespoon tomato paste.

- 1 tablespoon brown sugar.

- Six large spinach wraps.

- ½ ripe avocado.

- One 15-ounce can black beans, drained and rinsed.

- 1 cup shredded Romaine lettuce.

- ½ cup chopped cherry tomatoes.

- ¼ cup chopped cilantro leaves.

- One medium lime, cut into six wedges.

How to:

In a medium bowl, put cayenne, paprika, turmeric, salt, and pepper. Mix and add chicken breasts. Mix together. Jacket on both sides. Jacket on both sides.

In a slow cooker/pressure cooker bowl, place chicken. Add vinegar, water, sauce Worcestershire, a paste of tomato, sugar.

Bake the chicken in the oven for 30 to 40 minutes at 350 ° C or at 165 ° C in internal temperature. Cook in a slow cooker or pressure cooker as guided. Shake the chicken with two forks and put the sauce in a bowl.

For 30 to 60 seconds, each tortilla in a pot over medium heat until it's moist. Spread each one over the entire surface with a thin slice of avocado.

Split the ingredients evenly among six tortillas in the center of the tortilla; add chicken, beans, lettuce, tomatoes, cilantro, and a lime wedge squeeze.

Place the two sides in the middle of the tortilla and then tilt it below the bottom half and cover the top half of the tortilla to make a close burrito seal.

Creamy Slaw and Veggie Wrap

You can have a delicious wrap with hearty whole grains in minutes that benefit cognitive health and mental agility. Thanks to their phytochemical substances and antioxidants, whole grains offer many brain benefits as well as anti-inflammatory protection, which has proven to be a slow cognitive decline. Do you get at least three portions of whole-grain a day?

The broccoli offers vitamin C, fiber, and beneficial B vitamins such as folate, which help heart health and also contribute to brain health. A daily serving of vegetables can protect against cognitive decline and memory linked to Alzheimer's disease. However, research shows that in this recipe, pulses such as the black beans protect against losing your mental sharpness.

INGREDIENTS:

- 2 cups broccoli and carrot slaw.

- ½ cup marinated artichoke hearts, chopped.

- ½ cup black beans.

- 3 to 4 sprigs fresh cilantro, coarsely chopped.

- One tablespoon extra-virgin olive oil.

- One tablespoon balsamic vinegar.

- 1 teaspoon Dijon mustard.

- Two tablespoons plain low-fat Greek yogurt.

- Salt and pepper to taste.

- Three 10-inch whole-grain wrap.

How to:

Place the slaw, artichokes, beans, and cilantro in a medium bowl, blend softly until mixed.

Stir in oil, vinegar, mustard, yogurt, salt, and pepper in a small bowl. Pour over the mixture of the slaw bean. Toss well coated together.

Place the wraps on a cutting board. On each tie, position 1/3 of the slaw. Roll up and serve. Serve them. Enjoy! Enjoy!

DINNER RECIPES

For a supper of dementia, prepare and make some quinoa into a stir-fry, sprinkling potato, leafy greens, and beans in olive oil. Schwartz said these leafy greens are filled with brain-enriching vitamins, antioxidants, and minerals. Select an extra virgin variety regarding olive oil, says Schwartz, who notes that there are monounsaturated fat and polyphenols that lead to lower cholesterol. Furthermore, it is anti-inflammatory, and "evidence shows that cognitive loss is linked to brain inflammation." Wash all of this with a glass of wine-red or white that proves to improve good cholesterol.

Stir-fries

Think Chinese cuisine. Slice the meat or poultry into small pieces, cut quickly into a hot pan, and add some sauce. Pre-sliced frozen vegetables and Chinese and Thai bottled sauces make this simple.

Basic chicken, snow peas, mushrooms, water chestnuts stir-fry for one

Sauce INGREDIENTS:

- 1/4 cup chicken broth.

- Two teaspoons rice wine.

- 1 1/2 teaspoons soy sauce.

- 1 1/2 teaspoons cornstarch.

- ¼ tsp garlic powder.

- ¼ tsp ginger powder.

- 3-ounce chicken breast, no skin or bones, sliced thin.

- ½ onion, sliced into ¼ inch wide pieces.

- 1 cup sliced mushrooms.

- 1 cup snow peas or snap peas.

- ¼ cup sliced water chestnuts.

How to:

Mix ingredients of the sauce, hold.

Heat a small amount of oil over high heat in a pot or wok

Add chicken to the pot, stir and cook until pink is gone.

Add onions, snow peas, mushrooms and stir until hot

Stir in the sauce until the sauce is thickened and all the ingredients are coated.

Stews

Crockpots or HotPot is natural for stews in a crockpot set. I consider that crockpots offer a more intense aroma than hotpots, and lowering the number of herbs is better.

Crockpot recipe:

- 1 lb. beef stew meat or tri-tip cut into 1-inch pieces.

- One onion, sliced into crescents.

- ½ pound mushrooms, sliced.

- 1 lb. bag of mini carrots.

- Four red potatoes washed and cut into 1-inch pieces with skin on.

- 2 cups beef or chicken stock.

- 1 bay leaf.

- ½ tsp cumin.

- ½ tsp thyme.

- ¼ tsp pepper.

How to:

Place it all in the crockpot. Cook on low for 6 to 8 hours. Add salt or pepper or other seasonings and taste.

Loaded rice

INGREDIENTS:

- 2 cups brown rice, cooked.

- 1 egg.

- One onion, sliced into crescents.

- 1 cup frozen peas.

- ½ cup sliced mushrooms.

- 1 cup snap peas, cut into 1-inch pieces.

- 1 tsp soy sauce.

- ¼ tsp garlic powder.

- Scramble the egg.

How to:

Put all ingredients but the rice in. Stir fry it until all the veggies are done Then add the rice and stir together

Mexican casserole

INGREDIENTS:

- 1 tbsp olive oil.

- 1 sliced onion.

- 1 sliced red bell pepper.

- One sliced Anaheim chili or hotter pepper, depending on your taste.

- One can nonfat refried beans.

- 1 cup cooked brown rice.

- 1 cup (or more) shredded cooked chicken from yesterday's roast chicken.

How to:

Preheat the oven to 350 ° C

Sprinkle the olive oil onion and peppers low, set aside.

In the casserole dish, non-fat cooled beans plate, brown rice, fajita vegetables, the night before grilled chicken and salsa. Bake in the oven at 350 ° C until heated. Add salad, tomato, and guacamole.

Pasta

INGREDIENTS:

Pasta is sauce noodles on top. Alfredo sauces do not follow MIND diet guidelines, but sauces based on tomatoes do.

Basic spaghetti meat sauce:

- 1 pound of extra-lean ground beef or ground turkey

- 1 tsp olive oil

- 1 onion, diced

- ½ to 1 lb. sliced mushrooms

- One large can chopped tomatoes, with juice

- 2 8-ounce cans tomato sauce.

- One small can chopped black olives.

- 1 bay leaf.

- 1 tsp dried basil.

- ½ tsp dried oregano.

- ¼ tsp cumin.

- ¼ tsp pepper.

How to:

Saute turkey or beef in olive oil, chop meat until it is crumbly fried.

Attach onion, cook before accountability begins

Add the champignons, mix, and cook until the champignons are heated.

Add all other ingredients, cook for at least 1/2 hour.

Pour over non-GMO fried whole wheat noodles.

Chicken Curry Salad with Ginger, Almonds & Grapes

INGREDIENTS:

- 2 cups chicken broth.

- 1/2 cup almond slivers, toasted.

- 1/2 cup mayonnaise (recipe below).

- 1 1/2 pounds skinless, boneless chicken breast.

- Five teaspoons mild curry powder.

- 1/2 teaspoon ground ginger.

- One tablespoon fresh lime juice, plus more to taste.

- One 6-ounce cup plain strained yogurt (like Greek or Icelandic).

- 1 teaspoon honey.

- 1 1/2 inches fresh ginger root, peeled and minced.

- One medium red onion, chopped (1 cup).

- One yellow bell pepper, cored and small diced.

- 1 1/2 cup seedless grapes, halved or quartered.

- 2 heads butter lettuce, leaves separated.

- Salt and pepper to taste.

How to:

Preheat oven to 350 F. Preheat oven. Clean, dry, and prepare all fresh fruits. Spread the almond slivers over a baking sheet in one layer and bake for 5-8 minutes (check after 5 min).

Combine chicken broth and 3 cups of water in a medium pot on medium heat. In low heat, add curry and ginger to a little skillet, occasionally stirring, toasty and fragrant, for 3 to 5 minutes. Place aside. Set aside. In the meantime, pat chicken breasts dry with towels of paper. When a liquid is simmering, add the chicken (the liquid should be covered), adjust the heat to keep the chicken simmering, if necessary. Cook for 7 minutes, uncovered. Remove from heat and cover until chicken is cooked for 20 minutes. Remove chicken from the pot and place it for at least 10 minutes on the cutting board.

Make the mayonnaise (see directions below) while the chicken is cooking, if done, and set aside in the refrigerator.

Combine mayonnaise, cream, lime juice, sweetheart, curry, cinnamon, and fresh ginger in a large bowl. Season with pepper and salt. To mix whisk. Add onion, bell peppers, grapes, and almonds, stirring gently into a coat (for this part, I used a soft spatula).

Dice in bite-size pieces (about 1/2-inch squares) when the chicken is cool enough to handle them. Fold the chicken gently into the mixture of main salad, using a soft spatula or hands.

Taste it. Taste it. If required, season with salt, pepper, and lime juice to taste. I finally added another tablespoon of lime juice to my liking.

Make Your Own Mayonnaise

INGREDIENTS:

- One pasteurized egg yolk (I like Davidson's Safe Eggs).

- One teaspoon fresh lemon juice.

- 1 teaspoon Dijon mustard.

- 1/2 cup olive oil.

- Salt and pepper to taste.

How to:

Egg yolk, lemon juice, and mustard together in a medium bowl until they are smooth and homogeneous. Season with pepper and salt. Drizzle slowly in olive oil, whisking vigorously to keep the mixture smooth. See, super easy, and tastes far better than store purchased.

Grilled Chicken with Mole Black Beans

Smoky, spicy black beans are the star of this show; with less effort, they give all the deep flavor of a classic mole. The MIND diet recommends a minimum of three to four portions of beans or lenses a week. You 're on your way to this goal with this dish in your repertoire.

INGREDIENTS:

- 1 1/2 pounds boneless, skinless chicken thighs (8 thighs).

- Two tablespoons ancho chile powder, divided.

- 3/4 teaspoon kosher salt, divided.

- Cooking spray.

- 1 (4-oz.) bunch scallions, trimmed.

- 1 tablespoon, plus.

- 1½ tsp. olive oil, divided.

- 2 cups chopped yellow onion (from 1 large onion).

- Three garlic cloves, minced (about 1 Tbsp.).

- 1/2 teaspoon ground cumin.

- 1/4 teaspoon ground cinnamon.

- 2 (15-oz.) cans no-salt-added black beans.

- 1-ounce bittersweet chocolate, finely chopped.

- One teaspoon instant espresso granules.

- 1 1/2 tablespoon, plus.

- 1½ tsp. red wine vinegar, divided.

- 1 cup very thinly sliced radishes (about 8 oz.).

- 1 cup loosely packed fresh cilantro leaves.

How to:

Sprinkle 1/2 tablespoon of chili powder with 1/2 teaspoon of salt. Let stand for 5 minutes. Let stand. Cover a spray cast iron barbecue pot or skillet and heat to medium-high. Add half of the chicken; cook until charred and cooked, about 4 minutes on each side (until a thermometer record 160 ° F). Transfer to a platform and cover with aluminum foil for warming. Save the rest of the food.

Place the scallions in the grill and grill, turning regularly, till charred and wilted, for 2-3 minutes. Move to the chicken pot.

Heat 1 tablespoon of oil over medium-high in a large bowl. Add onion and garlic, cook for 3 to 4 minutes, occasionally stirring until tender. Add cumin, cinnamon, and chile powder to 1 1/2 tablespoons. Cook, constantly stirring, 30 seconds. Drain the boobs and rinse one can. Add dried beans, chocolate, and espresso to the blend of onion; combine the rest of the beans with the mixture. Bring to a fryer and cook until sauce is slightly thickened about 5 minutes. Stir occasionally. Add 1 1/2 tablespoons of vinegar, and 1/4 teaspoon of salt remaining.

Toss with the remaining 1 1/2 teaspoons of oil and vinegar radishes and cilantro. Divide the mixture of beans, chicken, scallions, and radish between four plates.

Chicken and Wheat Berry Bowl

Brain boosting grains and a lean grilled chicken have a sparkling vinaigrette, sweet blueberry, and nice walnut crunch. Throw in farro or quinoa for the wheat beers, or some other whole grain.

INGREDIENTS:

- 3/4 cup uncooked hard wheat berries (5 3/8 oz.).

- 12 ounces French green beans (haricots verts), trimmed and cut into 2-inch pieces.

- Cooking spray.

- 2 (8-oz.) boneless, skinless chicken breasts.

- 1 1/4 teaspoon kosher salt, divided.

- 1/2 teaspoon black pepper, divided.

- 1/4 cup olive oil.

- 1/4 cup red wine vinegar.

- 1 1/2 tablespoons chopped fresh tarragon.

- Two teaspoon Dijon mustard.

- 2 cups fresh blueberries (10 oz.).

- 1/2 cup chopped toasted walnuts.

How to:

Hold a large pot of boiling water. Remove the wheat berries, reduce the heat to medium and cook for 45 to 50 minutes until tender. Stir in green beans and cook for 3 minutes. Drain the wheat and beans and rinse them with cold water until they are fresh. Transfer to a bowl. Transfer.

Cover a spray cast iron barbecue pot or skillet and heat to medium-high. Sprinkle the chicken with 1⁄2 salt teaspoon and 1⁄4 pepper teaspoon. Add the chicken and grill to 160 ° F, approximately 5 minutes per side. Transfer the chicken to a cutting board and leave for 5 minutes to rest before cutting.

Meanwhile, whisk the remaining 3⁄4 teaspoon salt, vinegar, tarragon, mouth, and 1⁄4 teaspoon pepper together.

In a bowl, add the blueberries, walnuts, and vinaigrette to the wheat berry mixture. Split the mixture evenly between 4 shallow bowls. Slice the chicken into the grain, then break the chicken into bowls.

Baked Tofu with Cilantro Pecan Pesto

This recipe highlights some really nice plant foods like tofu made from soybeans and made into an easy-to-slice cake. Tofu is a full protein food containing all the essential amino acids your body needs every day. Moreover, you get a lot of important minerals like iron, calcium, and magnesium for about 90 calories per 1/2 cup (check the list of calcium and/or magnesium sulfates ingredients) and potassium – all of which are nutrients that keep your blood pressure under review and bode well for your brain.

Dressed in cilantro pesto, pecans, extra virgin olive oil and cloves of fresh garlic, this dish has a health effect. Cilantro contains virtually no calories and gives a fresh and unique taste. It is filled with essential oils and vitamins A and B. Moreover, the small leaves contain antioxidant flavonoid compounds that prevent damage to your cells and improve cognitive health.

In the meantime, pecans carry fats that are good for you and an abundant source of vitamin E, a powerful antioxidant that protects the brain. Nuts such as pecans can slow down age-related deterioration by reducing oxidative stress and inflammation, according to the MIND Diet.

INGREDIENTS:

- One package extra-firm tofu, cut into cubes.

- 2 cups cilantro, leaves, and stems.

- 1/2 cup pecans, chopped.

- 1/4 cup extra-virgin olive oil.

- 1/2 cup Parmesan cheese, grated.

- 1 large garlic clove.

- Dash of salt and black pepper to taste.

How to:

Preheat 400 F oven. In a medium bowl, place the tofu and set aside. Add cilantro and pulse to a food processor. Add pecans and pulse until they are combined; add oil and pulse a few times. For a period of 15 to 20 seconds or until well mixed, add cheese, garlic, salt and pepper, and puree.

Put the pesto over the tofu and mix gently until the tofu is coated well. Place in the oven or cooking sheet in an oven. Place in the oven. Bake 20 minutes, test, and gently toss tofu. Placed another 10 minutes in the oven. Repeat until the tofu is golden and bubbling brown on the edges. Remove from the oven and add a few tofu chunks to the tomato soup or over angel hair pasta on the top of a green salad.

Grilled Peach Avocado and Arugula Flatbread

It's a comfy bed to a multitude of nourishing toppings — vegetables, fruits, nuts, seeds, beans, chicken or turkey breast, fish, tofu, and yogurt sauce all work.

This formula uses whole flatbread grain (or naan bread if you prefer), which is a good dietary fiber and is a whole grain. There is scientific evidence that whole grains are cognitive benefits that lead to higher tests in infants, gradual cognitive loss, and memory intact in the middle ages and beyond. The role of whole grains in brain health is millions of years old.

The arugula also provides cognitive security in this recipe. Leafy greens are a major component of the MIND diet, as their nutrients, including folate, vitamin E, carotenoids, and flavonoids have shown to support better cognitive skills. Furthermore, the extra virgin dressing based on olive oil gives the brain some natural antioxidants and anti-inflammatory compounds to remove harmful proteins from the skin. The extremely "healthy" fat avocado can also help to reverse or delay cognitive declines.

INGREDIENTS:

- Two tablespoons extra-virgin olive oil.

- Two tablespoons balsamic vinegar.

- 1 teaspoon Dijon mustard.

- One dash of salt and black pepper.

- One large ripe peach washed and sliced.

- Two large whole-grain flatbreads or naan bread.

- 2 cups arugula, washed and dried.

- ½ large ripe avocado, cut into small chunks.

- Two tablespoons grated parmesan cheese.

How to:

Grill preheat to 400F. Whisk together oil, vinegar, mustard, salt, and pepper in a small bowl. Brush dressing vinaigrette onto fishing slices. Place them on the heated barbecue. Top the grill and allow for 1 to 2 minutes of peaches to cook. Flip over for another minute and cook. Disable grill. Disable grill.

Put flatbread on the grill to heat on each side for 30 seconds. Remove from the barbecue.

Place the rooster on any flatbread. Layer grilled peaches and avocado pieces, equally distributed on top of each, and sprinkle with parmesan. Drizzle and serve the rest of the vinaigrette.

Spicy Ruby Red Salsa

This recipe includes red tomatoes and red peppers, with red ingredients, plus fiery, smoky spices – cayenne and smoked (Spanish) paprika.

This salsa offers numerous of brain health nutrients. Were you aware that a portion of vegetables protects against cognitive deterioration every day? Coloring your plate will make a year and a half younger for your brain!

Cherry tomatoes offer a great nutritional bang for very few calories, with around 25 calories per cup. Tomatoes can keep inflammation at bay when combed with immune-enhancing vitamins A and C and folate. Moreover, in this recipe, the peppers double on vitamin C and potassium. This recipe also provides antioxidant strength from curcumin with a touch of ground cumin.

INGREDIENTS:

- 1 cup cherry tomatoes, coarsely chopped.

- ½ cup red peppadew peppers, quartered.

- One tablespoon, yellow onion, minced.

- One tablespoon extra-virgin olive oil.

- 1 teaspoon ground cumin.

- ⅛ teaspoon cayenne pepper.

- ⅛ teaspoon smoked paprika.

- Juice from ½ lime, cut into two wedges and squeezed.

- 1 pinch of kosher salt.

How to:

In a medium cup, mix all ingredients. Mix well and eat. Eat.

Pomegranate Mandarin Basil Champagne Spritzer

Excellent fresh ingredients-fresh grenades, mandarin oranges, and basil are at heart. I can imagine wanting to subscribe to the basil rosemary for an earthier fall scent, but my basil plant remains powerful and smells great. No good cocktail is overly sweet, so you've come to the wrong place if you're looking for that. This cocktail is gentle, smooth, and has a hint of herbal. There are true flavors, no sugar added to the mask, or weak ingredients.

INGREDIENTS:

- ¼ cup of water.

- One medium pomegranate yields a cup pomegranate aril, plus extra arils to use as garnish - keep this reserved to the side; keep some membrane, pith and peel reserved,

- One seedless mandarin orange, quartered and then each quarter halved.

- 1 cup fresh loosely packed basil leaves, rinsed, dried and roughly chopped or torn.

- Optional: 1 oz orange liqueur (I used Patron Citronge orange liqueur premium reserve 80 proof).

- Optional: 1 mandarin for peels of zest as garnish.

- Optional: basil leaves for garnish.

How to:

Heat the water for medium heat until it cools down. Add grenade arils, diaphragm, pitch, and peel.

Mix with a large wooden spoon, carefully crushed arils, around 2-3 minutes, so that juice is released without splattering.

Remove the mandarin pieces and proceed to cook and smash with a wooden spoon back for around 2-3 minutes to release the juices.

Continue to stir, smash arils, and mandarin pieces, when needed, some 3-5 minutes longer before they are reduced to a syrup consistency.

Add basil and mix to add aromas for about a minute.

Squeeze for a half cup of liquid.

Add orange liqueur to stretched liquid and remove it if used.

Refresh until use.

Add a tablespoon of a champagne flute, champagne top, fresh pomegranate arils, basil leaves, mandarin zest. To serve. Love the outing.

Chicken Curry Salad with Ginger, Almonds & Grapes

INGREDIENTS:

- 2 cups chicken broth (I used a store-bought organic chicken broth, but this is a great way to use any homemade broth you may have laying around in the fridge or freezer).

- 1/2 cup almond slivers, toasted.

- 1/2 cup mayonnaise.

- 1 1/2 lb. skinless, boneless chicken breast.

- Five teaspoons mild curry powder.

- 1/2 teaspoon ground ginger.

- One tablespoon fresh lime juice.

- 6 oz cup plain strained yogurt.

- One teaspoon honey.

- 1 1/2 inches fresh ginger root, peeled and minced.

- One medium red onion, chopped.

- One yellow bell pepper, cored and small diced.

- 1 1/2 cup seedless grapes, halved or quartered – pick your favorite, I used a mix of red, green, and black California table grapes.

- 2 heads butter lettuce, leaves separated.

- Salt and pepper to taste.

How to:

Preheat oven to 350 F. Preheat. Clean, dry, and prepare all fresh fruits. Spread slivers of almond on a baking sheet in one layer and bake for 5-8 minutes until lightly browned.

Combine chicken broth and 3 cups of water in a medium pot on medium heat. At low heat, add the curry and ginger powder to a saute pot and occasionally stir for 3-5 minutes until toasted and fragrant. Set aside. In the meantime, pat chicken breasts dry with towels of paper. When the fluids are cooked, add chicken (the fluid should be covered) and adjust the heat to keep it dry if necessary. Cook for 7 minutes, uncovered. Remove from the heat, and cover until chicken is cooked for 20 minutes. Remove chicken from the pot and place it for at least 10 minutes on the cutting board.

Make the mayonnaise during the cooking process and put it in the refrigerator during cooking.

Combine mayonnaise, cream, lime juice, sweetheart, curry, cinnamon, and fresh ginger in a large bowl. Season with pepper and salt. To mix whisk. Add onion, bell peppers, grapes, and almonds to coat (in this part, I used a soft spatula).

Dice into bite-size pieces (~1/2-inch squares) when chicken is cool enough to handle. Fold the chicken gently into the mixture of main salad, using a soft spatula or hands.

Taste it. Taste it. If required, season with salt, pepper, and lime juice to taste. I finally added another tablespoon of lime juice to my liking.

Snack recipes for the **MIND** diet

Pita chips

Cut pitas into triangles.

Place on baking sheet.

Bake at 374 degrees for 5 to 7 minutes, till crisp.

Dip recipes

Hummus

INGREDIENTS:

- 1 clove garlic.

- 1 (19 ounces) can garbanzo beans, half the liquid reserved.

- Four tablespoons freshly squeezed lemon juice.

- Two tablespoons tahini (sesame seed paste).

- 1/4 teaspoon.

- Black pepper to taste.

- Two tablespoons olive oil

How to:

Dump all in a mixer or food processor except olive oil. Mix or heat until pasty. Put in a pot, make a depression and position the depression of olive oil

Baba ghanoush

INGREDIENTS:

- Two medium eggplants (about 3 lbs. total), roasted.

- 1/3 cup tahini from light seeds, not "dark tahini."

- Three cloves garlic roasted (or one raw clove, minced).

- Juice of 2 whole fresh lemons, or more to taste.

- 1/2 tsp cumin.

- 1/4 tsp salt or more to taste.

- Black pepper to taste.

- Two tbsp extra virgin olive oil.

How to:

To roast the aubergine:

Rinse the eggplants and poke them with a fork in many locations. To capture fall, cover a bakery sheet with foil or parchment. Do not use parchment if the eggplants are broiled using this board.

Broil the eggplant for a smoky taste, turn every 2 minutes, and the skin starts to smell smoky. (If the eggplant isn't in your broiler, it can be charged over a flame – use two long-sleeved forks or large tongs to keep the eggplant safe.

Place eggplants on the sheet in your middle oven rack. Bake until soft at 375 degrees 25 to 30 minutes. Cool up until your hands catch it – usually ten to fifteen minutes.

In a medium bowl, combine tahini, garlic, lemon juice, cumin, salt, and pepper as you wait for the eggplant to cool up.

Split the roasted aubergines. Remove extra liquid and remove it. Scrape the flesh out of the skin and put a mixture of Tahini into the bowl. Sprinkle the eggplant with the tahini mixture.

Drizzle the top with the olive oil and dip into it. (Or, if you make a later event, store the egg mix and add olive oil on top.) Keep up to 5 days in a refrigerator.

Other snacks for the MIND diet (dried berries, nuts, and olives):

- Almonds.

- Blueberries (dried).

- Cashews.

- Cranberries (dried).

- Hazelnuts.

- Olives.

- Pecans.

- Sunflower seeds.

- Walnuts.

Alzheimer's Prevention Recipes

MIND combines the best of the DASH and Mediterranean diets to minimize Alzheimer's risk and promote the health of the brain. Start to make healthy choices today!

Gluten-Free Ramen Noodles with Sesame Garlic Greens Recipe

The MINd diet emphasizes the provision of leafy green vegetables such since the Swiss chard, as they include folate, vitamin E, carotenoids, and flavonoids, which are associated with a lower risk of dementia and cognitive decline. The highest protective effect on brain health has been a daily dose of leafy greens — equivalent to one and a half years younger! Furthermore, the entire grains in this dish provide brain-healthy nutrients, vitamin E, and other antioxidants, which can help to preserve the functioning of your brain.

INGREDIENTS:

- One millet and brown rice ramen noodle cake.

- 1 cup Swiss chard, rinsed and coarsely chopped.

- 1/2 cup marinated artichokes hearts, diced.

- 1/4 cup carrots, shredded.

- 1 tablespoon sesame oil.

- One tablespoon low-sodium soy sauce.

- Two teaspoons freshly squeezed lemon juice.

- One large garlic clove, finely minced.

- Two teaspoons toasted sesame seeds.

How to:

Add two cups of water to a large pot and put it on the stovetop over high heat. Take a rolling boil and gently fall into the ramen pot. Allow it to cook for a minute, gently separated with a bucket. Turn heat to a gentle boil, allow to cook, occasionally stirring for three minutes. Drain in a sink colander.

In a large bowl, put cooked ramen. Chard, artichoke, and carrots. Toss in chard. Whisk butter, soy sauce, lemon juice, and garlic together. Drizzle over vegetables and ramen. Gently toss. Gently toss.

Divide into two bowls ramen and vegetables. Top each with its seeds of sesame. Enjoy! Enjoy!

Peanutty African Chickpea Stew

This meatless stew is full of nutrients and gives you a taste that will keep you happy and fulfilled for hours.

Spices include cinnamon, cumin, and cayenne pepper with a rich base of peanut butter. Sweet potatoes, chickpeas, and kale include filler and potassium, vitamins, and antioxidants that minimize blood pressure.

This African chickpea stew is fast and easy to make so that 45 minutes or less can be a dinner on the table.

INGREDIENTS:

- Two teaspoons olive oil

- Three cloves garlic, minced

- 1/2 medium onion, diced.

- 1 stalk celery, diced.

- One small sweet potato, cubed.

- 1 cup low sodium vegetable stock.

- 2/3 cup creamy natural peanut butter.

- 1 1/2 teaspoons ground ginger.

- 1 teaspoon ground cumin.

- 1/4 teaspoon cayenne pepper.

- One can (15-ounce) low sodium chickpeas, drained and rinsed.

- One can (15-ounce) low sodium diced tomatoes.

- 1 bunch kale, chopped.

- Chopped peanuts (for chopping).

- Cilantro (for chopping).

How to:

Heat oil over medium heat in a large bowl. Add garlic, onion, celery, and sweet potato and cook until celery and onion are softened.

Mix in the stock of tomatoes, peanut butter, ginger, cumin, and cayenne. Mix well. Mix well. Add chickpeas, kale, and tomatoes.

Turn heat down and cook, covered, until sweet potato is tender, about 20 minutes.

Sweet and Spicy Tofu and Jalapeno Pad Thai

This plain, enhanced version of an Asian classic blows your mind by enflaming your senses with a hint of warmth from jalapenos. Besides, it is a low-fat vegetarian alternative with the main source of protein tofu. It also provides anti-inflammatory effects from whole garlic cloves and healthy fats from crunchy peanuts on the rice noodles. The MIND diet requires nuts to eat most days — partially because they are a rich source of vitamin E, a nutrient that protects the brain, at least five times a week.

This dish also provides a good base to add a variety of vegetables. This vegetarian pad thai suits well in a brain-healthy menu with the MIND diet based on vegetables — with a regular service at least showing benefits from cognitive decline. Sprinkle in leafy greens to give it a special boost!

INGREDIENTS:

- 1 tablespoon peanut oil.

- Two garlic cloves, minced.

- One small jalapeno, seeds and membranes removed, minced.

- 1/2 cup mushrooms, sliced.

- One package tofu drained and cut into cubes.

- One package pad thai rice noodles.

- 1/4 cup lime juice.

- 1/4 cup low-sodium soy sauce.

- 1 tablespoon honey.

- pinch chipotle crushed red pepper.

- 1/2 cup peanuts, coarsely chopped.

- 1/2 cup carrots, shredded.

- Two tablespoons cilantro.

How to:

Place a wok or deep casserole on the stovetop over medium-high heat and add butter, garlic, peppers, mushrooms, and tofu. Sautes the tofu before browning and softening of vegetables.

Prepare noodles as directed in the package. Add cooked noodles with tofu and vegetable mixture to the wok or pot.

Whisk together lime juice, soy sauce, honey, and crushed pepper in a small cup. Pour the tofu and vegetables over it. While still over the heat, mix together. Remove when heated thoroughly.

Divide the noodle platter between six bowls. Sprinkle each with peanuts, carrots, and cilantro, if needed.

Homemade Vegetarian Lo Mein

This version of classic Chinese Lo Mein is a shock full of veggies, whole grain noodles, and vegetable protein. Brown rice and millet ramen noodles are sprinkled with a simple mix of veggies and a sweet and savory sauce.

The tastes flow well and have digestive benefits: fresh, unpasteurized cider vinegar and stomach calming properties of ginger include probiotics. Your brain also benefits from a variety of vegetables.

INGREDIENTS:

- Two brown rice and millet ramen cakes.

- Two tablespoons low-sodium soy sauce.

- Two tablespoons sesame oil.

- Two tablespoons agave nectar.

- One tablespoon raw, unpasteurized apple cider vinegar.

- One tablespoon fresh ginger, peeled and diced.

- One teaspoon Sriracha (hot chili pepper sauce) (optional).

- 2 cups stir-fry vegetable mixture (snow peas, carrots, bell peppers, onions, broccoli, and cabbage).

- 4 ounces firm tofu, patted dry and cut into cubes.

How to:

Prepare the ramen noodles following the package instructions.

Whisk soy, sugar, agave nectar, vinegar, ginger, and sriracha in a small cup, if used. Add to another large bowl of vegetables and tofu. Sprinkle with the sauce on top and toss until well coated.

Add vegetable and tofu in a large wok or pot over medium-high heat on the stovetop. Cover and heat for 10 minutes, occasionally stirring. When vegetables start to soften, they 're ready.

Add noodles to the mixture of vegetables and toss lightly. Remove from the stove and drink warm while still.

Pan-Seared Salmon with Mediterranean Quinoa

The Mediterranean diet is famous for its richness in fruit, vegetables, entire grains, fish, and healthy fats, while salmon is not originally from the Mediterranean; the flavor profile and nutrient content pairs beautifully with dietary characteristics.

In this pan-sear salmon with Mediterranean quinoa, the salmon is rich in heart-healthy, anti-inflammatory omega-3 fatty acids. Olive oil and olives add a heart-healthy bonus, with a little saturated fat with just the right flavor from the feta cheese. Quinoa, spinach, and sun-dried tomato fiber from whole grains can help reduce cholesterol, blood sugar, and digestion. All these ingredients make a safe and warm meal in a single bowl.

INGREDIENTS:

- 1/4 cup black olives.

- 1/4 cup sun-dried tomatoes.

- 1/4 cup fresh parsley.

- 1 clove garlic.

- 1/2 cup quinoa, dry.

- 1/2 pound (8 ounces) wild Alaskan salmon.

- 1/8 teaspoon black pepper.

- 4 cups baby spinach.

- 1 tablespoon olive oil.

- 1/4 teaspoon dried basil.

- 1/8 teaspoon salt.

- 1-ounce feta cheese.

How to:

Chop olives, tomatoes, and parsley dried with sunshine. Peel and a thin clove of garlic. Place aside. Set aside.

Cook quinoa according to the instructions of the package.

Put your salmon dry with a paper towel while the quinoa is cooking. Rub each slice with a small amount of olive oil and sprinkle with black pepper.

To medium-high heat a pot. Add the salmon skin side up once hot. Cook for three minutes, then turn over and cook for another three minutes.

During cooking, heat your olive oil and garlic in a separate pot over medium heat. When dry, add a few minutes of baby spinach and sauté until wilted.

Mix olives, sun-dried tomatoes, pearls, basil, and salt when your quinoa is finished. Last blend feta cheese.

Serve the quinoa and spinach with the salmon on top side by side. Enjoy!

Simple Vegetarian Spinach Lasagna

Nothing like lasagna can alleviate a longing for a creamy, dreamy meal. This Italian classical bend with its base of vitamin C-rich tomato sauce, which is filled with carotenoid lycopene, with a strong dose of veggies in the layers.

Full of leafy green spinach, this dish is good for your brain health since a portion of veggies has been eaten every day to prevent cognitive decline. Spinach is loaded with iron and calcium to improve the body's total wellness.

INGREDIENTS:

- One package no-boil lasagna noodles.

- Two 28-ounce cans tomato sauce.

- 1/8 teaspoon kosher salt.

- 1 teaspoon oregano.

- Two cloves garlic, finely minced.

- One 15-ounce container part-skim ricotta cheese.

- 1 cup part-skim mozzarella cheese, grated.

- 3 cups raw baby spinach leaves.

How to:

Preheat the 350 F oven.

Pour the tomato sauce into a saucepan on the stovetop over medium heat. Salt, oregano, and garlic are added. Bring to a light boil, lower the heat, and cook for a couple of minutes. Occasionally stir.

Put a layer of tomato sauce on the bottom of a 9x13 pan. Place a noodle layer above, covering the bottom of the tub. Dress the noodles with ricotta cheese, cover with spinach and top with mozzarella and a small ladle full of sauce. Repeat the layers to the top of the bowl. Sprinkle with mozzarella cheese in the final layer.

Bake for 45 minutes in the oven, or until golden brown is bubbly on top of the cheese.

Take out of the oven and cool 10 minutes before serving.

Creamy Vegetarian Pumpkin Cauliflower Soup Recipe

It gets no better than pumpkin soup unless you add cauliflower. Both of them are jam-packed with Phyto (plant) nutrients that protect your brain and body from chronic diseases.

Nutrients support the entire body: vitamin A and vitamin C help to prevent the common cold, and the cruciferous cauliflower confounds allow the brain to boost memory. However, pumpkin 's rich orange meat provides loads of carotenoids that are antioxidants to protect your body and brain from daily stress harm.

Smooth and creamy, this soup tastes like fall, with a mixture of musk and cloves. These spices offer the soup with their powerful aromas, a plethora of flavors, which lie on their buds and penetrate your senses for a feeling of well-being that warms your mind and body on a cold day.

INGREDIENTS:

- 1 tablespoon canola oil.

- One medium yellow onion, diced.

- Two 28-ounce cans pumpkin puree.

- One medium head of cauliflower, cut into small florets.

- 2 1/2 cups low-sodium vegetable broth.

- 1 teaspoon salt.

- 1 teaspoon black pepper.

- 1/2 teaspoon ground cloves.

- 1 teaspoon ground nutmeg.

- One teaspoon fresh tarragon, chopped.

- 2 1/2 cups low-fat (2% fat) milk.

- 1 teaspoon lemon juice.

How to:

Place the oil in a large stockpot over medium heat on the stovetop.

Attach the onions and allow for translucent cooking (around 5 minutes).

Attach the pot and mix. Remove. Five minutes of heat.

Add chocolate and broth; cover. Cover. Cook until cool (approximately 15 minutes) begins to soften.

Incorporate herbs and spices (salt through tarragon). Stir well and give another 10 minutes to cook.

Puree the mixture directly in the pot, using an immersion (hand-held) blender.

Add milk and mix well once smooth. Add the lemon juice, add a final mixture, and serve soft.

Easy Egg McMuffin-Style Sandwich

This version has unique anti-inflammatory properties — the eggs are scratched with turmeric, a spice found to prevent inflammation in the body. The eggs also have a generous protein aid: 12 grams! Also, new basil is thrown into the flavor, and nutrition improves egg scramble.

Avocado slices are nestled between the nooks and crannies of entire wheat, to give a smooth, good, fat boost plus plenty of potassium. This simple sammie will fill you and fuel your body every day.

INGREDIENTS:

- One whole-wheat English muffin, toasted.

- Cooking spray.

- Two large eggs scrambled

- One teaspoon ground turmeric.

- 1 teaspoon garlic powder.

- Two fresh basil leaves, sliced.

- 1/8 teaspoon kosher salt.

- 1/4 of a small avocado, sliced.

- One thin slice beefsteak tomato.

How to:

Put in the toaster per half of the English muffin. Enable toast until the edges are slightly browned and crisp.

Apply a spray of cooking spray to a small pot on the stovetop over medium-low heat. Scrap eggs with turmeric, garlic, basil, and salt in a small cup. Put in the heated pot. Scrap the eggs gently and smooth with a spatula. Remove from heat. Remove from heat.

Place the scramble on half of the muffin toasted. Cover with slices of avocado and tomatoes.

Fill with the muffin portion. Serve warm while.

Sesame Garlic String Bean Almondine

This one-pan dish is a balanced alternative to the conventional green bean saucepan. The green beans provide a portion of vegetables. According to MIND 's dietary studies, it helps protect your brain from cognitive decay up to 1 1/2 years younger!

Sprinkling with soft almonds contributes to good fats, vitamin E, and calcium. This contributes to reducing oxidative stress and inflammation. They also supply food, folate, and flavonoids to your brain and body. It means that cognitive loss has slowed down, and survival has improved in the long term.

In this dish, the garlic and onions also save the brain from cognitive decay — after all, it is good for your heart, too.

INGREDIENTS:

- 1 tablespoon sesame oil.

- 1 garlic clove, minced.

- ¼ large white onion, minced.

- 2 cups green beans, washed and trimmed.

- ½ freshly squeezed lemon juice.

- ¼ cup raw, slivered almonds.

- A pinch of kosher salt.

How to:

In a medium saute pan, add oil and garlic over medium-low heat. A minute saute. Saute. Add the onions and saute for a further minute until the onions are translucent and browned around the edges.

Toss the beans in the orange. Mix, cover, and allow a few minutes to cook. Remove from time to time and allow a few more minutes to cook and steam under the cover.

Add the lemon juice, almonds, and salt to cook. Saute until green beans start to smooth. Remove from heat. Remove from heat. Toss and serve in bowls or plates.

Smoky Baked Bean Medley

The beans are good for your overall health because they fill you with fewer calories, which are good for weight management, cholesterol, blood sugar, and blood pressure. Eating beans have been shown to delay cognitive loss daily. In other words, beans are protecting your brain against aging!

In addition to the fiber, this dish offers the ruby red goodness of cooked tomato sauce loaded with the lycopene antioxidant. They are improved to a balance of taste and gut-friendly bacteria by cheap, unpasteurized apple cider vinegar, and alloy shallots from the vegetable family, which are perfect for cancer prevention and keep your heart safe. Honey adds a light hint of a naturally sweet flavor that boosts your brain 's energy.

INGREDIENTS:

- Two 15-ounce cans tri-bean blend (kidney, pinto, and black beans), rinsed and drained.

- Two 8-ounce cans tomato sauce.

- One tablespoon extra-virgin olive oil.

- 1 small shallot, minced.

- One teaspoon smoked paprika.

- ½ teaspoon garlic powder.

- One tablespoon raw, unpasteurized apple cider vinegar.

- 1 tablespoon honey.

How to:

Preheat 350F oven. In an oven-safe bowl, add beans and tomato sauce. Stir gently until mixed.

Add oil to a small saucepan on the stovetop over medium-low heat. Twenty seconds of heat; add shallots. Sprinkle until transparent for a few minutes. Remove from heat. Remove from heat.

Add cooked shallots and tomato sauce to the dish. Add the paprika, garlic powder, vinegar, and sweetheart. Remove gently until mixed together.

Place in the refrigerator. Refrigerator. Bake and mix for 30 minutes. Bake for 15 to 30 minutes to bring the aromas together. Remove and serve from the oven.

Brain Sharpening and Nourishing Recipes

Here are a couple of delicious and healthy recipes, including brain stimulation, that will keep you sharp. I put together these recipes, including desserts, smoothies, sides, food, or something to satisfy all of you. So, friends, we 're going to dig in!!

Immune Boosting Green Smoothie

INGREDIENTS:

- 1 large handful Spinach.

- One thumb-sized piece of Ginger.

- 2 Medjool Dates.

- 2 Oranges (juiced).

- 1/2 Lemon (juiced).

- 1/4 tsp Turmeric Powder.

- A quick, immune-boosting green citrus smoothie. Perfect for taking on the go on a morning, you're in a rush!

How to:

Juice the citrus fruit and add the spinach to the mixer. Put the dates in place and add the peeled ginger and turmeric. Blend at high speed to smoothness. Serve immediately. Serve immediately.

Pan-Seared Orange Mustard Salmon

Pan-sewn orange mustard salmon – easy, healthy, 15-minute marinade dinner. Healthy food foods, pasta, rice cauliflower, or asparagus.

INGREDIENTS:

- 1 teaspoon butter.

- 3 Salmon Filets.

- 1/2 cup orange juice.

- Zest of 1 Orange.

- One tablespoon ground Mustard.

- One teaspoon Light Soy Sauce.

- 1 teaspoon honey.

- One teaspoon of rice wine vinegar.

- Salt to taste.

- Sesame Seeds for topping.

How to:

In a cast-iron skillet, heat butter and add the skin of the salmon filets down. Cook the salmon 4-5 minutes until the skin is very crooked.

Whisk in a small bowl orange juice, zest, mustard, soy sauce, sweetener, vinegar, and salt and add to the plate. Bring it to a fast boil and fry the sauce for 2-3 minutes before it grows thick. Flip the salmon gently and cover it with sauce (I like spooning the sauce over it). Serve immediately with sesame seeds. Serve.

Pomegranate & Dark Chocolate Bites

INGREDIENTS:

- 2 1/2 cups pomegranate seeds.

- 5.25 ounces (150 grams) high-quality dark chocolate.

- 1 tablespoon of sea salt.

How to:

Sprinkle a single layer of pomegranate seeds across 12 muffin cups.

In the microwave, melt the dark chocolate in a small bowl. Verify also that it is not smoking.

In a piping bag or plastic bag, add the melted dark chocolate. Snipe off the end so there can be a small stream of chocolate.

Pip a chocolate pattern across the grenade seeds. Attach another layer of grenade, more chocolate, and the final layer of a grenade.

Finish on each pomegranate chocolate bite with a pinch of sea salt.

Cool for at least an hour before serving. Serve immediately after removing from the fridge.

Cooked Ripe Plantains

Cooked plants are the easiest but a great treat. When cooked, they are very healthy. It tastes good, smooth, and easy to digest when cooked. The cooked mellow plantains are one of the solid foods we give to children aged 8-9 months. They are also very beneficial for adults. When cooked, the nutritional value of plantains changes, but for good. Here we give you two healthy methods for cooking mature plantains.

INGREDIENTS:

- One Yellow Plantain Perfectly ripe.

- Water for steaming.

Equipment:

- For Microwave method.

- Microwave safe bowl with a lid or plate.

- For Steam Cooking.

- Steamer with lid.

How to:

We can cook the ripe plantains by two methods.

1. Microwave

Wash in cold water the plantain.

Cut the plantain's two ends.

Place it in a healthy bowl with a microwave. The plantains can be cut in half to fit into the dish.

Cover with the lid or plate loosely.

Cook on high power for 5 minutes.

Check if it is soft and cooked like potatoes.

If not fully cooked, you can turn the plantain and cook for another 1-2 minutes.

Let the heat dissipate covered for 1 minute.

Transfer to a plate. Transfer to a plate. Remove the peel. Remove the peel.

Cut it into small disks and enjoy it.

2. Steam Cooking

Wash in cold water the plantain.

Fill the steamer with water and bring to a boil.

Inside the steamer, place the washed plantain. Cover with lock. Cover with lid.

Cook until soft for 10-15 minutes.

Transfer to a plate the cooked plantain.

Peel and enjoy the fur.

Recipe Notes Recipe

Do not close the lid tightly when microwaving. If the deck is close, the steam within the bowl cannot escape and is harmful. Lock the lid during the microwave.

The exact cooking time depends on the power and maturity of your microwave. If you are over-ripening, you will need less time to cook.

Summer Love Salad

INGREDIENTS:

- ½ cup macadamia nuts halved.

- 1 tsp caster sugar.

- 1 tsp salt.

- 2 cups spinach washed.

- 1 tsp olive oil.

- Eight asparagus spears.

- 12 strawberries halved.

- Six bocconcini quartered.

- ¼ cup mint chopped.

- 1 tsp balsamic glaze.

How to:

In a frying pan, put the macadamia nuts over medium heat. Fry until brown, then add salt and sugar. Remove for about 1 minute or until the sugar has dissolved and turns dark golden brown. Put nuts on a baking paper sheet to cool.

In a large bowl, place the spinach and toss with olive oil.

Remove the ends from the asparagus spears and woody pieces. In a bowl, put asparagus in a little water and microwave for 1 minute or until the green and tender are clear. To stop the cooking process, run under cold water. Diagonally slice.

Spinach top with balsamic glaze almonds, asparagus, strawberries, mint, and drizzle.

Idli

INGREDIENTS:

For the batter:

- 3 cups idli rice this is not same as raw rice we use in day to day cooking.

- 1 cup of raw rice normal rice/pachaiarisi.

- One ¼ cup whole urad dal white color (ulutham paruppu).

- 1 1/2 teaspoon fenugreek seeds methi seeds/vendhayam.

- Water as required.

- Salt to taste.

How to:

Add idle rice and raw rice in a bowl. Rinse them underwater once, and soak them insufficient water. Put whole urad dal and fenugreek seeds in another cup. Add soaking water. For a minimum of 6 hours to a maximum of 10 hours, rice and dal should be soaked separately.

After soaking, rinse the rice and dal once again 2 to 3 times separately.

Add urad dal with little water to the grinding boiler first and grind until it is smooth and fluffy. It could take 30 to 50 minutes based on your grinder and the amount of the dal used. Add water between grinding times in very small quantities (every time about a tablespoon of water). Scrap the sides during grinding so that all Dal grains are evenly ground. The quality of the urad dal batter is one of the secrets to soft idlis. The batter must be very smooth and fluffy (after melting volume doubles)

Remove the dal into a large bowl once done and set aside.

Then, without washing the grinder, add soaked rice and melt until the rice turns into a smooth batter, adding a little water each time. Take the urad dal batter into the same saucepan.

Mix the batter together with a stainless-steel spatula. For a good 8 to 10 hours, set aside for fermentation. Overnight hopefully.

You will see the batter doubling its volume the next day and rising up well. Mix well with a spatula, add salt and mix again. That's it. That's it. This is the ideal idli/dosa batter.

The batter consistency for idlis must be thick in order to become soft spongy idlis. Don't add water to the batter if you intend to hurry. And if you want to use this dose batter, take a part of the required water batter, add a very small water mix, and test if you have the right water consistency, then use the dose batter.

I use the aluminum idle cups to make idles in a traditional way. And I use a wet cotton tissue instead of grating the pan with oil, onto which I pour the idli batter for 10-12 minutes and gently remove it from the tissue.

In these traditional idle steamer pans, Idli turns out to be very fluffy, soft, and big. Serve hot and steaming fluffy idlis with sambar tiffin, chutney cocoon, chutney onion-tomato spiciness, chutney mint. Or just serve idlis with idli podium powder with few drops of warm ghee (clear butter).

NOTES:

The rice and urad dal ratio are the most important aspect of making idli batter. I've always used a ratio of 4:1.4. I use 1 1/4 cup whole urad dal for 4 cups of rice (3 cups of idli rice, 1 cup of raw rice).

ALWAYS use the entire urad dal while the batter is being made. The broken ones are not the same results for you.

The soaking time for both urad dal and rice should be at least 6 hours. A well-soaked rice and urad dal give a good smooth batter.

Fermentation is another key factor in getting the perfect idli or dosa. Make sure the batter is kept moist naturally for 8 to 10 hours. If your kitchen isn't warm enough in the season, you may need to ferment for a lot longer than 10 hours, or heat your oven to the lowest temperature, putting the batter into the oven with oven lights.

If the color of your idle rice is red, you get idlis that are somewhat reddish. I love my idlis, so I use only white idlis in color. I love my idlis.

I mentioned the recipe for a common batter, both idli, and dosa. Make the batter a little thin while making doses and use it. But don't add water to the batter to make idlis. As mentioned above, the Idli batter should be thick.

The thin crisp, nice browned doses are from the same batter as fenugreek seeds are added in urad dal. Don't skip that. Don't skip that.

Super Green Tea Antioxidant Smoothie

This Super Green Tea Smoothie is made of spinach and matcha green powder. Protein, vitamins, and antioxidants are loaded!

INGREDIENTS:

- 1 cup unsweetened almond milk.

- ½ banana, peeled.

- 1 cup loosely packed fresh spinach leaves.

- 1 cup strawberries, hulled.

- ¾ cup ice.

- 1 serving vanilla protein powder (1/2 to 1 scoop depending brand).

- ½ teaspoon matcha powder.

How to:

In a blender, add almond milk, bananas, spinach, strawberries, salt, protein powder, and matcha powder.

Puree at high speed until the ice is not completely smooth, around 45 seconds.

Homemade Yogurt

You can easily make a healthy and naturally fermented yogurt recipe at home. There is no yogurt maker to make delicious, homemade yogurt.

INGREDIENTS:

- 2 cups of whole milk.

- 1.5 tsp. plain yogurt store-bought or from the previous batch.

How to:

In a bowl outside the refrigerator, keep the plain yogurt (unflavored) to bring it to room temperature. This releases the bacteria. That's the word.

In a deep and thick bottom pot, bring the milk to a boil.

Remove the heat and keep cool.

The milk temperature should be between 110 and 115 Fahrenheit (43 to 45 Celsius).

You may follow this method if you don't have a thermometer. The milk should be warm enough to make your finger burn. The milk should be warm to keep the bacteria alive.

In the bowl, add the warm milk to the yogurt. Mix well with a spoon to evenly distribute the food.

Cover the bowl with a rag. Do not use a narrow deck or cover the bowl tightly.

Let it restless in a warm place, preferably an oven (when it is cold) for up to 12-14 hours or until it is thick and tasteful.

Cool the yogurt to obtain a thick texture.

Serve as required. Serve as required.

NOTES:

Save a little yogurt from the previous batch for the next batch.

Check for 12 hours of yogurt thickness. If not, keep it untouched before you get a thick yogurt.

The fermentation process may take longer during the first batch. It depends on weather conditions, crop quantity of active bacteria, milk type, protein content, etc. In warm conditions, the fermentation process is usually faster.

Anti-Inflammatory Lemon Turmeric Tonic

INGREDIENTS:

- 4" fresh turmeric root (or two teaspoons dried turmeric).

- 3" fresh ginger root.

- Juice of 2 organic lemons.

- 1/4 teaspoon fresh ground pepper.

- 4 cups coconut water or filtered water.

- Optional: Sweetener of your choice like raw honey or stevia.

How to:

Cover with a towel or parchment and scrape the skin off the turmeric with a knife. Point the tip of the spoon to the top of the root and just slowly push down, and you'll see how simple the skin is. Use gloves or other towels to avoid staining your hands. The spoon also works to remove the skin from the ginger.

In a high-speed blender, put turmeric, ginger, lemon juice, pepper, and water and blend together. (Alternatively, all the ingredients

can also be juiced). Add sweetener and taste if desired. Keep
chilled.

RECIPE TIPS

Food storage

Some people keep their staples in this way: If you create several soups or stews, store their main ingredients together. It's quick to grab all of them and put them in your morning slow cooker to have a meal ready for you in the night. So canned tomatoes go rather than all in one place into your soup area, your pasta sauce, and your stew area.

Freeze leftovers in meal-size quantities.

You can freeze leafy greens without the trouble of blanching after rinsing them if you are to use them in a few weeks.

Cooking and eating tips

If you like sticky brown rice, use short grain brown rice, add half cup of liquid, and cook half an hour, and automatically release in a press cooker.

Have a bread meal at breakfast and a sandwich made from 2 slices of whole-grain bread at lunch to get your three portions of whole grain.

You can use berry powders and green leafy powders to add smoothies and soups to get enough fruits every week.

Powder sum equivalent to 1 cup of fresh fruit or vegetables

If you choose to substitute a certain quantity of powdered fruit or vegetable for the fresh one, the quantity of powder to be eaten is equivalent to one cup of new.

Sweet Potatoes – 1 cup.

Collard Greens – 1 tablespoon.

Blueberries – 7 tablespoons.

Spinach – 1.5 teaspoon.

Carrots – 2 tablespoons.

Tomatoes – 1 tablespoon.

Kale – 1 teaspoon.

The diet of the Mediterranean diet and DASH is known to prevent and eliminate 4 of the big deaths in America: cardiovascular disease, obesity, cerebrospinal stroke, and cancer. There is evidence that they can also minimize the occurrence of Alzheimer's disease and slow down memory.

The MIND diet was developed by taking a closer look at all the elements of certain diets that are obviously beneficial to health in general and that Western diet ingredients have a detrimental impact on health. In people who follow such diets, they were associated with memory tests and Alzheimer's disease.

The findings showed that unique food requirements support improve brain health.

THE MIND AS A VEGETARIAN

If you are a vegetarian, you will need to tweak the MIND diet to ensure adequate consumption of brain-protective compounds like omega-3 fatty acids, vitamin B12, and protein.

Omega-3 Fatty Acids

Omega-3 fatty acids from fish are EPA (eicosapentaenoic acid) and DHA (docosahexaenoic acid), whereas only ALA (alpha-linolenic acid) from the plant sources is a precursor not effectively converted into DHA and EPA within the body.

The biggest downside of a vegetarian MIND diet will be the loss of DHA omega-3 fatty acids that are highly correlated with the decreased Alzheimer's disease levels.

For vegetarians, two omega-3 alternatives are omega-3 oil and perilla oil algae.

Algae oil supplements are an option because of their high DHA content, which is comparable in fish.

Perilla oil is obtained from perilla seeds and is capable of stopping or improving Alzheimer's. In rodents, mice, and nerve cells, perilla oil ALA had similar cognitive effects to DHA. While chia seeds in ALA are also strong, cognitive impairment in mice has not improved.

B12

In B12, animal proteins are strong, an important vitamin not widely found in herbal foods. For DNA synthesis and nerve and blood safety, B12 is essential. In clinical and observatory research, Low B12 is associated with decreased memory and increased levels of Alzheimer's disease.

Vegetarians can supplement or supplement MIND-diet with plant-based foods high in B12, including nori algae and shitake mushrooms.

PROTEIN

The full spectrum of protein amino acids is important for the proper function and functioning of the brain. Vegetarians who omit all animal-based proteins from the MIND diet will require compensation for a weekly loss of around 75 g of protein.

Many vegetable foods with a high content of protein include:

Tofu (3oz): 14g.

Quinoa, uncooked (½ cup): 9g.

Pumpkin seeds (⅓ cup): 33g.

Almonds (⅓ cup): 18g.

Tempeh (3oz): 17g.

Black beans, uncooked (½ cup): 13g.

Lentils, uncooked (½ cup): 16g.

RECIPES

Vegan ABC Chocolate Pudding with Pistachios and Orange Zest

INGREDIENTS:

- Three ripe medium bananas, peeled.

- Two ripe medium California avocados, peeled and deseeded.

- ½ cup unsweetened cocoa powder.

- 1 tsp vanilla extract.

- ¼ tsp chili powder.

- ½ cup pistachios.

- Zest from 1 medium orange.

How to:

Pudding: Combine all ingredients until smooth, except for pistachio and orange zest. Cover and let it cool for 1 to 2 hours, or until fully chilled.

Prepare pistachios: oven to 350 F. Preheat oven. Toast pistachios for 3 minutes on the baking sheet. Remove and bake for a further 3 minutes. Let it chop coolly and grossly—store until ready to serve in an airtight jar.

Serve: Divide into eight dessert bowls, top with pistachios. Serve. Divide a whole orange medium (or two, if you love orange zest) into cups.

Sunshine Vegan Breakfast Salad

The bright and tangy, yet creamy and rich avocado-lime dressing are contrasting with this sunset-inspired breakfast salad with its aromatic sweet mango, buttery avocado, and raw almonds. The bed of red butter baby lettuce provides a soft foundation. Every bit of this unique breakfast salad is a great day for you.

The plant protein prevents blood sugar even in the almonds, and polyphenols, antioxidants, vitamins, and minerals provide nutrition for your mango and blueberries. Recent studies into brain wellbeing, leafy greens, nuts, berries, and olive oil have helped protect the brain from cognitive loss – so here this morning, they all enjoy.

INGREDIENTS:

- 1 medium mango.

- Two large limes.

- 1 medium avocado.

- Ten sprigs of cilantro.

- 1 tsp olive oil.

- 5 oz pre-washed baby red butter lettuce (about 6-8 cups, loosely packed).

- 6 oz organic blueberries (about 1¼ cups).

- ½ cup almonds.

- Salt and pepper to taste.

How to:

Wash all goods and dry them.

Peel the mango, slice off the mango for two big cheeks, and cut thinly in the longitudinal direction. It ends up being loosely packed around 1 and 1/4 cups.

Remove the green of lime and avoid the bitter white pith; thin (or use a zest) for 1 tsp of the lime; set aside.

To make 3 tbsp juice, cut the limes in half and the juice. Save the remaining lime half.

Cut the avocado in half, throw out the seed and peel the skin away. To avoid browning, using leftover lime halves to squeeze lime juice over the avocado.

Make dressing. Render the clothing. Compose half the avocado, lime zest, lime juice, cilantro, and olive oil in a high glass with a hand blender (or a small mixer/food processor) and mix until smooth. Season to taste with salt and pepper. Makes approximately 3 oz of dressing.

Combine salt, mango, blueberries, and almonds with dressing in a large bowl. Help with plastic gloves.

Slice in width the remaining half of the avocado.

Divide the salad and about 1-2 cups in each bowl into four bowls. Cover with slices of avocado. Add extra cilantro to garnish if desired.

Tri-Color Vegetarian Egg Rolls Recipe

This recipe transforms the traditional, fried, meat-filled finger food into a baked, vegetarian version employing a Chinese staple, the egg roll, into a healthier plane. Each egg roll is packed with green and red chocolate and carrot slaw and offers a powerful cruciferous punch for brain health. The slaw is tossed with a light sauce, which adds a minimal flavor.

The paper-thin egg roll wraps are each filled with only 55 calories. Loaded with veggies, they are a large low-fat fiber and plant-based goodness conduit for a healthy mind and body.

INGREDIENTS:

- 12 egg roll wraps.

- 4 cups cabbage and carrot slaw.

- Two tablespoons low-sodium soy sauce.

- 1 tablespoon sesame oil.

- 1/4 teaspoon ground ginger.

- 1 teaspoon raw honey.

- One tablespoon rice wine vinegar.

- Optional: 1/4 cup sesame oil for brushing.

How to:

Preheat to 350F. Preheat oven. Put the egg roll wraps on a lined baker's sheet in the shape of a diamond (with pointed edges on top and bottom).

In a medium bowl, put the slaw. In a small bowl, whisk the soy sauce, oil, ginger, honey, and vinegar. Drizzle over slaw sauce and sprinkle until covered.

Spoon the middle of a wrap with a small spoonful of the slaw mixture. Fold the lower corner over the filling; tightly roll to cover the filling. Fold both sides, left and right, against the fill; roll over the rest of the corner to the tip. Place the roll flap on the baker's side down. Brush oil tops, if desired. Oil. Bake until the tops are lightly browned 15 to 20 minutes.

Rosemary Vegetarian Eggplant with Pistachio Nuts

This recipe includes brain-healthy, low calorie, and carbs ingredients such as eggplant, a good source of fiber and potassium. Moreover, vitamin E pistachios contain healthy unsaturated fats, proteins, and carotenoids lutein and zeaxanthin, which are good for cell health overall.

Extra-virgin olive oil adds hundreds of powerful antioxidant and anti-inflammatory compounds and healthy fats to the mind-enhancing mix. Note that the extraction of oil after cooking helps preserve its health-enhancing properties, as heating it too high can damage its delicate nutrients on a plant basis.

INGREDIENTS:

- One medium eggplant washed and cut into small chunky pieces.

- ¼ cup shelled lightly salted pistachios, coarsely chopped

- 3 sprigs fresh rosemary, washed and finely diced.

- One tablespoon smoked paprika.

- One tablespoon extra-virgin olive oil.

How to:

Preheat oven to 400 ° C. Throw all ingredients into a medium oven-safe bowl except olive oil. Mix well together until mixed. Cook in the oven for 45 minutes to 1 hour.

Check every 20 minutes and stir. Once the breadcrumbs are soft and browned, remove from the oven and allow 5 minutes to sit. Drizzle with oil and gently toss to cover.

Easy Vegan Zucchini Noodles with Avocado Pesto

INGREDIENTS:

- Two zucchini ends cut off, and cut into spiral noodles with a spiralizer or shredded with a grater or food processor.

- 1/2 avocado peeled.

- One tablespoon pine nut plus extra for garnish.

- 1/2 clove garlic.

- Juice from 1/4 of a lemon.

- 1/8 teaspoon sea salt.

- Fresh ground black pepper.

How to:

Make the zucchini "noodles" with a spiral, scratch, or food processor and set aside.

In a food processor or blender, mix the remaining ingredients and scrape the sides accordingly.

Mix the pesto with the courgettes and tops if desired with additional pine nuts.

MIND DIET BENEFITS

The key goal of researchers in creating the MIND diet was to reduce the risk of Alzheimer's disease (AD). It is estimated that approximately half-million Americans younger than 65 years have some type of dementia, including Alzheimer's disease, according to the Alzheimer's Foundation of America.

Morris and her team have been performing MIND diet experiments for almost a decade, working with a group of 923 seniors. The results showed that diet reduced the risk of Alzheimer's in participants who carefully adhered to the diet by as much as 53 percent. According to the Rush University Medical Centre, it also supported 35% of those who adopted the diet reasonably well.

The study also found that the longer an individual followed the MIND diet, the better the individual was protected from developing Alzheimer's. In March 2015, the study's findings were published in Alzheimer's & Dementia: The Alzheimer's Association Journal.

For another report, Morris's team compared the MIND diet with DASH and Mediterranean diets head-to-head. The results with the other two diets were similar to those with the MIND diet alone. According to Rush University Medical Center, high adherence to the diets decreased the incidence of Alzheimer's by 39% of those who adopted the DASH Diet and 54% of those who adopted the

Mediterranean Diet. Nevertheless, the two other diets did not benefit much if they could be identified as mild rather than strict.

"One of the most interesting aspects here is that people who have adhered to the MIND diet only mildly have a decreased risk for AD," said Morris in a press release of Rush University. "I think people are going to be inspired."

Different studies have shown that increasing the Mediterranean diet and the DASH diet has health benefits in other areas too. For example, in one study, people who followed the DASH diet experienced a 3-month decrease in blood sugar levels. In that study, scientists believed that the decrease is due to higher probiotic consumption than the diet prescribed. DASH may also help decrease the blood pressure by a handful of points in just two weeks, according to the Mayo Clinic, while systolic blood pressure may decrease by eight to 14 points over time.

Another research, published in April 2010, found the Mediterranean diet to reduce weight and cholesterol, triglycerides, and blood pressure across diets. The Harvard School of Public Health and the Cambridge Health Alliance have researched 780 male firefighters and found that the Mediterranean-style diet has been related to lower cardiovascular risk factors.

HOW DOES THE MIND DIET DIFFER FROM OTHER DIET PLANS?

While the MIND diet does not include exercise directly, daily physical activity can also help prevent cognitive deterioration, as movement increases blood flow to the brain and helps provide nutrients to brain cells. According to the Alzheimer's Research and Prevention Foundation, regular physical activity can actually reduce the risk of Alzheimer's disease by up to 50%. Exercise, in conjunction with the MIND diet, may also provide additional memory loss security.

The MIND diet also varies from other common diets because calories are not counted, and food groups are not excluded. Vanessa Rissetto, RD., a nutritionist based in Hoboken, New Jersey, says the paleo and ketogenic (or keto) diets are more restrictive than the MIND diet. Both popular diets minimize whole grain consumption, and paleo omits milk as well. The MIND diet, on the other hand, is not too restrictive and highlights the rise in food intake with cognitive benefits. As a result, you also have a balance between enjoying your favorite foods, sweets, and wines.

Keep in mind that while this plan is especially helpful to those who are at increased risk for Alzheimer's disease or dementia, to benefit from this diet, you do not need to be older or have a family history of the disease. Kerkenbush says, "Anyone will benefit from the MIND diet because of its overall balanced eating style, and there are no adverse side effects.

Since this diet is plant-based and contains several different types of food, whether you cook meals at home or eat out is typically simple to stick with. Nonetheless, despite this diet, the focus on berries and nutrients can contribute to a slightly higher food bill than other packaged, less nutritious snacks.

TIPS FOR FOLLOWING THE MIND DIET ON A BUDGET

The MIND Diet has shown excellent results in memory development. However, the reliance on nuts, berries, and plants will make it a costly diet. Using these tips simultaneously to secure the brain and budget.

EAT FROZEN BERRIES INSTEAD OF FRESH

Fresh berries can be a drain on the budget, and they can not be accessed during the year in many parts of the world. Purchase instead of frozen fruits and add them to smoothies or yogurt, bake them into muffins, wheat pancakes or waffles, or heat them with water to enjoy the oatmeal in a balanced coating.

USE CANNED OR DRIED BEANS

The MIND Diet suggests every other day one serving of beans or legumes. Canned beans are cheap, easy to reach, and fill. Make sure that you have a choice of lentils, red and white beans, chickpeas, or kidney boots in your shopping list, so you don't get shrugging.

Consider joining a wholesale supply store

Wholesale companies like Costco are subject to a subscription fee, but they are a great place to shop for food in bulk. Three portions of whole grains a day and one portion of vegetables (plus green foods) are included in the MIND Diet. Store them on brown rice and pasta and test the frozen vegetables. A big bag of frozen broccoli costs just under $5 and is new in quality.

Buy chicken legs and thighs

Two portions of poultry are recommended every week by the MIND Diet. When shopping in food, many people hit the chicken breasts immediately, believing that they are healthier. But the quality of the thigh and the breast meat is very close, and the thighs are much cheaper than chicken breasts. Better still, buy an entire chicken, which is the best way to eat poultry per pound.

Look online for deals on nuts

Unlike fruits, nuts are another part of the MIND Diet that may add a dent to the budget for your weekly meals. Skip the store and search for bulk sales online. You can buy an almond supply for around $10 for two weeks. Mind that the dosage of nut is only 1 oz. Serve two to five days a week.

Make sure you're following the recommended portion sizes

You just need to eat 1 oz of nuts a day to get a quarter. Weigh one time out to see how tiny it is: 1 oz equals about 20 almonds, 17 cashews to 14 walnuts.

BUY IN BULK AND FREEZE

See a lot about chicken thighs but don't think that until they spoil, you should eat them all? Don't allow that to stop you from stealing. Buy a lot and add to the freezer instantly what you won't eat.

LOOK FOR CHEAPER VARIETIES OF FISH

When shopping for fish, the cost of the well-known varieties is simple. Cod, halibut, and sea bass are all good, but if you eat them once a week, they can burn a hole in the pocket easily. Consider cheaper options such as dorados, porgies, and sardines. Don't be delayed until you've cooked them before – several recipes for these lesser-known forms of fish are available online.

DON'T WORRY IF YOU CAN'T FOLLOW THE DIET EXACTLY

In my research, only those who adopted the MIND diet decreased their risk of Alzheimer's by 35%. When finances are a war, concentrate more on what you can do.

CONCLUSION

I love this diet — it's a blend of two super-nutrient-rich diets that give anti-inflammatory, cardiac, and brain health benefits. The emphasis on fruits and vegetables, healthy fats, less processed and refined foods is a perfect way for most of us to eat every day.

While some memory deficits are common as you age (forgetting where you placed your keys, you won't find a word at the tip of your language), severe memory loss is not a guaranteed thing. By focusing on what you eat, you can keep your mind healthy and raising the risk of severe memory deteriorations. Your diet, along with some other lifestyle factors, will influence the way your brain functions and develop your logical thinking skills such as learning something new, processing important information, addressing problems, managing complex tasks, and critically thinking.

The effect of diet on memory can be achieved surprisingly quickly. The memory will increase as quickly as 1 hour after a protein drink and go down one hour after a glucose drink. In addition, a low-glycemic breakfast (with a slight decrease in glucose after peaks) with better verbal memory in the course of the morning than a high-glycemic breakfast (with high-grade glucose peaks and rapid decreases).

Nutrition has an effect on brain function; however, well beyond the hours of consumption. Yes, for years, the food we consume may have a positive or detrimental impact on our brain health.

Early work has shown that diets in the Mediterranean and DASH have a link to better brain health, perhaps as a result of enhanced cardiovascular functioning. Researchers wondered, however, whether these results can be strengthened by mixing the most beneficial Mediterranean and DASH diets with foodstuffs known to enhance brain health and foods, which should be minimized because of their negative impact on brain health. The MIND (Mediterranean-DASH Delay Intervention) Diet was thus established. The findings of retrospective MIND Diet studies were groundbreaking.

It's not necessary — or even a good idea — to wait for signs that your memory drops until your brain health is discussed. By eating like your mind, you can maximize your brain's working and think abilities rely on this – because they do.

That said, it's always a good idea to consult with your doctor before you start a restrictive diet.

Do Not Go Yet; One Last Thing to Do

If you enjoyed this book or found it useful, I'd be very grateful if you'd post a short review on Amazon. Your support does make a difference, and I read all the reviews personally so I can get your feedback and make this book even better.

Thanks again for your support!

9 798692 568526